Dedicatio

Dedicated to every women in the world, never forget how beautiful and worthy you are. You have the power within. If it's in your head, it's a dream, if it's in your heart it's a passion, and then you can have it in your hand, reality.

Dream, Passion, Reality.

Foreword

It often feels that we are given every reason to fail in life. Poor upbringings, unforeseen circumstances, and broken relationships are holes that can feel impossible to climb out of. Social obstacles like prejudice and misogyny add another weight to our shoulders, only increasing the list of excuses at our disposal. At the end of the day, it seems the easiest option is to simply give up and blame our circumstances for our shortcomings.

This mentality makes it just as easy to hunt for excuses. When things don't go our way in life, it is commonplace to look for something, or someone, to take the blame for instead of ourselves. One excuse I hear a lot is "I'm too old". Not only is that a lie, but it is disrespectful to your true capabilities! Many iconic and successful figures, including Arianna Huffington, Vera Wang, and Julia Child, didn't even get started until they were over forty. If you think that success in life just "isn't for you" due to circumstance, abilities, or age, you could not be more wrong. Do not sell yourself short, as you are capable of incredible feats. "Don't Wait in the Wings" knocks down the notion that you have to be young to chase your dreams and find joy as a woman. It is never too late for success and to be an inspiration to the younger generations. Don't just sit back and watch as the people around you follow their dreams and find what truly fulfills them. The world spins with or without us, and it is up to YOU to change your mindset. As women, we know very well that nothing is handed to us, so we need to capitalize when opportunities present themself. Be aggressive, dream big, and follow those dreams.

Of course, this is way harder said than done. The pressures of the world to fit in with culture and society are ever-present and can make it seem there is a pre-destined path of monotony for us all to walk. Gender roles from centuries past still rear their heads in our lives and apply even more pressure and expectations. Growing up, we all had expectations placed upon us by family. Some parents are adamant they know the path their children will walk and try to influence it in the worst ways possible. When we don't meet these sometimes impossible expectations, it is easy to let the guilt overwhelm us until all we see in the mirror is a failure.

I personally want you to know that you are far more than the expectations unfairly placed upon you. Life is not about what is expected of you, but how you overcome the obstacles that come your way. We all need to live life on our own terms and find joy and success in personal victories. Success is relative, and small feats to one individual can be the thing of dreams to another. I know women whose parents expected lengthy and expensive doctorate degrees to decorate their walls. And yet, simply attending college, the first in their families to do so, was a huge success in itself. Do not let others define what makes you feel happy or successful. Instead, embrace what gives you fulfillment. Do what YOU love, and not strictly what makes others happy. It is your life and yours alone. These two ideas often go hand in hand, and in finding fulfillment you will often improve the lives of people around you too. It is not selfish to take care of yourself. In fact, to truly serve your friends and family, you must make yourself right first. Obviously, we can't abandon our roles as mothers, wives, and friends, but we all need to take the necessary time to embrace success and joy in our lives.

The book you hold in your hands empowers women through information and gives them permission to be true to themselves, and not to the expectations placed upon them. “Don’t Wait in the Wings” is a collection of stories from a team of successful and mindful women who have lessons to share about self-fulfillment when the whole world feels against us. Each story is a personal journey and highlights how each author kicked down their respective obstacles to ultimately find personal success.

Stripped down to its basic themes, “Don’t Wait in the Wings” is about authenticity. Too often we go through life putting on different faces for different groups of people. Giving a good impression is so important to us that we are willing to let the pressures of our expectations mold us into women who do not resemble our true selves. We need to stay authentic, and not shy away from what makes us happy. What is life without fulfillment? “Don’t’ Wait in the Wings” tells the story of what happens when women decide to stop conforming and start searching for success. So dream big, and do not resist that inner fire within you. Each and every woman reading this is capable of incredible accomplishments and will find joy if it is sought. Take the time to care for yourself, and to find what brings you fulfillment. Along the journey, you will become happier, and will positively affect the lives around you. Feed your inner fire, and break through every obstacle that comes your way. I guarantee you can be successful; it will just take a little elbow grease to get there.

Contents

Follow Your Passion

By Rachel Withers

"Allow your passion to become your purpose, and it will one day become your profession."- **Gabrielle Bernstein**

There was never a doubt in my mind that I was going to be a dancer when I grew up. I loved dancing when I was a young girl. I'd prance around the kitchen with the radio on and dance. I'd watch performances of *Swan Lake* and *The Nutcracker*, joining in with the prima ballerinas as they twirled on stage. I'm sure that my parents saw it as a phase I would grow tired of, as little girls often do, but they soon realized that even though I was young, my love of dance trumped the rest of my hobbies. When the opportunity came for me to begin to train professionally in ballet, I was quick to join a class. It was no easy feat and training my body to perform the graceful moves of the ballerinas I'd watch perform took time and effort. Yet, I persisted because dancing was something I wanted to do. As I grew older, my passion for dance continued to burn. I was able to put into words why I liked to dance, how it made me feel happy to dance in my class's studio. I loved the feeling of my dance costumes brushing against my skin as I twirled across a stage, I adored the weightlessness of leaping into the air, and I was enchanted by the different routines that my class performed. Even though I was still young, I couldn't imagine my life without dancing.

With my higher education, my love for dance morphed into the attempt to fulfil the dreams I had as a little girl; to be able to become a prima ballerina and dance on stage for thousands of people to see. I took an opportunity to train with the Royal Ballet School and took my passion to a whole other level. My imaginary ballets as a young girl were fully realized and I performed in places that I had only watched on television. That feeling was one that I knew I'd never forget. I got my bachelor's degree in Performance Arts and decided to pursue my dancing in a more formal setting. As time continued on, my body was beginning to show the signs of slowing down. I don't think many people realize the toll that rigorous physical activity has on your body, which leads them to being surprised when men and women retire from those kinds of careers before they reach the age of forty. Retiring from professional dancing didn't stop my love for it, but I began to focus on other things in my life a bit more than my passion. I fell in love with someone and got married and, soon after, we had two children. I began to focus on my home life more and more, letting my love of dance fade more and more into the background of my life.

It was at the point when I became a mother that I felt as though my passion had burnt out. I could remember how excited I was when I was a little girl, just dancing around my house to the radio, but that excitement didn't seem to want to show itself now that I was older. Not to say that I was unhappy where I was with my life; I had a loving husband and two beautiful children that I couldn't have been more proud of, but something seemed to be missing. I did most of my work from home, my focus being more on my family life and job instead of what I used to love.

I began to notice things about myself that I wasn't happy with. I had gained weight and after two pregnancies, I didn't get back into a regular exercise routine. I was self-conscious about my looks and just how age was affecting my body. The years of dancing had taken their toll on my muscles, but without regular stretches or exercise, I was unable to bend like I used to. I couldn't move as quickly and my joints hurt as the years went on. There were times where I wanted to try and do a bit of dancing again, but either I was too tired or I didn't have enough time.

As my time as a mother went on, I found that I just identified with the roles I was in now. I was a wife and a mother and it didn't seem like there was any room for me to be anything else. With my dancing career behind me after putting in so many years of time and effort into it, I didn't feel like I could call myself a dancer anymore. My sense of identity caused some friction with my relationship with my husband. I knew that he was trying so hard to understand where I was coming from and wanted to do what he could to make me feel better, but no matter how hard I tried and no matter what help he gave, I still felt like a part of me was closed off, unable to meld with who I was. My self esteem grew worse and I didn't feel like I was the same woman that my husband had married. He assured me otherwise, but it didn't stop the intrusive thoughts that I was too fat and too slow to still be the same woman that used to leap into the air without getting winded.

"The things you are passionate about are not random, they are your calling." **-Fabienne Fredrickson**

One day, my youngest daughter and I were walking along a busy street. She was just like me when I was younger, always moving and dancing around. I encouraged it when we were at home or in an open space, but I didn't want her to dance her way into something dangerous. On that particular day, she was a bit too antsy and ended up nearly running into traffic. I never moved so fast in my time as a mother; I can still remember the feeling of the pavement under my feet, jostling my bones and muscles as I ran to grab her before she made it into the street. When I got her back onto the pavement, she was crying from being snatched up so quickly and I was completely and utterly out of breath. I think I ended up nearly collapsing onto the pavement with her in my arms. I remember the sheer exhaustion I felt as I hugged my little girl close to try and calm her down. Even though I was sweaty and still struggling to get my breath back, I remember thinking that the near death experience probably counted as my exercise for the day. After getting my daughter back home and collecting myself, it hit me how far I was from my prime as a dancer. I would have been able to grab her without even breaking a sweat. I wouldn't have felt pain in my joints from the sudden burst of adrenaline and I would never have felt like I had the wind knocked out of me. The realization that I was so far from what I had been when I was dancing was a wake-up call for me. I knew that

I had to make a change if I wanted to see a positive change in my self esteem and in my home life. Sure, I was past my prime as a ballerina, but that didn't mean that I couldn't do something to get myself back into form.

It took a lot longer than I had hoped to get back into a routine of stretching and remembering some of the dance exercises I used to do. I worked hard to create a new routine that allowed me to get back some of my dancing. As I stretched and worked my muscles, I remembered the burn I felt when I first had to stretch in my beginner ballet class and how tough it was. I was brought back to myself as a little girl, excited to be learning about dancing and willing to put up with the pain and aches in order to succeed. The passion I had for dancing slowly began to rekindle itself, finding its way to incorporate itself into other parts of my life without disrupting my own routine or my family's. My husband noticed how I was getting in shape and took some time out of his routine to stretch with me. My kids would attempt to join in, giggling when they came up with their own ballet moves when they couldn't replicate mine. I watched in delight as the pounds fell away each time I stood on a scale and I found that my stamina increased so that I wasn't winded while trying to keep up with my kids. My mood improved with my weight loss. I loved the fact that I was able to dance again and work my body into familiar positions that recalled a much different time of my life. I can remember looking in the mirror a few months after my daughter's close call and feeling happy with the woman that I saw there. I didn't look like I did when I was at the peak of my career and there was still some flabbiness to my stomach, but I was satisfied with what I looked like. I smiled at my reflection, a true smile that wasn't forced or put on just for show. I felt genuinely happy and a part of me wondered why I hadn't done this sooner.

My husband and kids weren't the only ones who noticed the changes in my mood and appearance. Friends I hadn't spoken to in years wanted to reconnect and, since I was more satisfied with my overall mood and appearance, I accepted after a few months of politely turning many of them down. When we'd meet, I'd get so many compliments on how good I looked, even though I wasn't dancing professionally anymore. I told my friends about what I had decided for myself and what I was doing to keep in shape while also continuing to do something that I loved. Many of my friends were excited for me, some of them commenting that they wished they had the time to get back into their dance routines as well. Those conversations were what sparked the idea for BalletBeFit and, after a bit of time, I was able to go back to those friends and help them get their own passions back. "I'll let you in on a little secret. We don't all love our jobs every day. And doing something you have passion for doesn't make the work part of it any easier...It just makes you less likely to quit." - **Kate Jacobs** If you told me that I'd become an entrepreneur and business owner when I was pursuing my dance career, I honestly don't know if I'd believe you. With how passionate I was with my dance career, I couldn't have imagined doing anything else.

Of course, life doesn't always turn out the way we intend. I lived my dream, then found further happiness with my husband and children. However, because of the loss of my passion, even that new happiness became something I struggled with. It was only by rediscovering my love of dance and shaping that love in a way that suited my life at the time that I was able to feel satisfied and content. Again, I didn't magically transform my body back to where it was at my prime, but just getting into better shape did wonders for my health and mood.

I feel that as we grow older and we have more responsibilities, we tend to place our passions on the backburner until those responsibilities are handled. We can get so caught up with our daily routines and new challenges that we may forget about our passions all together and the interest in them burns out. Throughout my career as a public speaker, I've found that this is the case for many people. Some men and women realize that they've begun to lose their passion for their favorite activity and don't bother to try and reignite that flame because they don't have the time. Others are more concerned with other aspects of their lives and feel that their passion would get in the way. I hate to say it, but I've met a few people who felt as though they needed to sacrifice their passion in order to get through their lives successfully.

Your passion is special and shouldn't have to be something that is forgotten to time. Because I had let go of my passion, I lost a part of my own identity. Understanding that my passion for dance couldn't just be left in the past helped me to remember why I loved it so much. I learned that I wanted to share my love of dancing with the world and, even if I wasn't able to do the things I could when I was younger, I could still translate that love into something that could show others.

BalletBeFit was the catalyst for me to showcase the techniques I had learned through my years of dance and help others to work towards their fitness goals by showing them my passion for dance. I knew my business wouldn't resonate with everyone, but those who had lost their love of dance were able to find it again through my program. It also helped me to further develop my own beliefs as to how to keep healthy while still wearing all of the hats that came with running a business and being a mother. I thought that I'd be satisfied after developing my new business, but I found that I wanted to do more. I studied coaching methods, working more through self-development thoughts and actions that could help people who lost their passions to regain them, and another part of my business took off. I began speaking to those who were in the same boat as I was; those who had lost their passion in some way, shape, or form. I wanted to show them that they didn't need to compromise with the way they lived their lives. They could still pursue their passions and loves without sacrificing them and instead shape them into something that they could utilize with their new routines.

"Too many of us are not living our dreams because we are living our fears."-**Les Brown**

There was a part of me that feared reigniting my passion. I knew there was something missing in my life, but my love of dancing should have been easy to identify as the solution. It should have been so simple to remember my passion for dance and reignite it, but I allowed other aspects of my life and career to overshadow it. When I started to practice my exercises again, a part of me was still unsure if I should be doing it. I was older, not as flexible as I once was, and getting back into a routine was hard to balance with the rest of my responsibilities.

The thought that plagued me the most was this: even if I got into better shape, would I still want to dance again? After so many years of focusing on other aspects of my life, would I still be able to feel the same passion for dancing that I had when I was younger?

The answer turned out to be a resounding yes. Sure, I needed to allow myself more time to get more flexible and remember the moves, but because my love of dance was my passion, I was able to bring it back into my life in a new form. I fell in love with it again, just like I had when I was a little girl, and that love continued to grow every day.

When coming up with a plan for my business, I could feel that fear creeping back into my life again. There were so many ways that my plans could fail and I didn't know if I could have contingencies for everything that could happen. Still, I knew I needed to take that chance because I loved what I was doing and it turned out more than alright once BalletBeFit was introduced to the world. Taking that chance was what allowed my passion for dance to ignite even further but helped to ignite other people's passions for dance as well.

"If passion drives you, let reason hold the reins."- **Benjamin Franklin**

The above quote is something that has resonated with me years after launching my business and working as an entrepreneur. As great as it would be for me to focus on my passion for dance the way I had when I was younger, I understand that I'm not able to go back to the way things were. When I was younger, I didn't have the responsibilities that I have now as a mother and a wife. When I was in training, I didn't have my other businesses to worry about or my family to care for. I needed to make sure that my passion stayed with me, but it needed to be reworked in order to fit into the life that I had made for myself.

I like to use the example of romantic comedy movies to illustrate how not to reignite your passion. There's always a character that's struggling with attempting to balance his or her life with their love of something they used to do. In many cases, that character drops everything to pursue their passion and the movies don't focus on the repercussions of those actions. When I realized that I needed to make a change in my life, I couldn't just leave my husband and kids to get back into my life as a dancer; it wasn't what I wanted to do and it would be unrealistic to think that I'd be able to pick up exactly where I left off before my retirement. My body doesn't work the way it used to when I was in my prime and I'm more prone to injuries because I was out of shape. And how could I ever think of leaving my family? I loved them with all my heart and just because I was missing my passion didn't give me the excuse to leave them in order to get it back. I needed to be reasonable with how I brought my passion back into my life. I had to be aware of what my body could handle and how much dancing I could do while still providing for my husband and kids. I used my dancing to get myself back into shape as an exercise routine, working it into my life without disrupting the other routines I had built after my retirement.

"The most powerful weapon on earth is the human soul on fire."-**Ferdinand Foch**

My passion for dancing allowed me to be where I am today and reigniting it allowed me to find a place for it in my career. I don't know where I would be now if I hadn't rediscovered it in a new form that fitted my way of life.

There were so many chances for my passion to burn out again and again, but I've kept it reignited after all of these years. Taking that chance to bring it back into my life made my life fuller and more complete. Just looking back on my time as a dancer didn't bring my passion back; I had to actively participate in its rekindling in order to have it conform to my way of life. My actions throughout my life paved the way for its resurgence and showed me that I still needed my passion to help make my life complete. The best piece of advice that I can give you is that you can't just wait for your passion to come back to you. Be an active participant in that rekindling, no matter what form it takes. Start writing in a journal to get back into writing. Find karaoke tracks on your favorite music services so that you can sing in the car or in the shower. Set some time out of your day to work on your art. No matter what it is that you enjoy, you need to take that first step to help you get your passion back.

My book is called *Don't Wait in the Wings* for a reason. There are far too many times in our lives where we can jump into a situation that provides us the inspiration to keep moving towards our goal, but most of us never take it. We end up standing to the side and watching as others take that leap of faith, wishing that we had the courage to do it ourselves. Through my experiences, I've learned that we always have just the type of courage to take that leap. Sure, it may not be an immediate change, but if you want to do something that resonates with you, you'll find that it just takes a few steps to dive in headfirst.

I'm also not saying that you need to be unprepared for this leap. Surprisingly, many of the people I speak to about going out onto their stage of life and taking a risk already have the tools and preparations they need to succeed. What keeps them from moving is the fear that they'll mess up or make a fool of themselves. As Shakespeare wrote, "All the world's a stage, and all the men and women merely players;" we find ourselves on the stage of life in front of a crowd of thousands of people who are waiting for our turn to perform. It's a scary thing to perform with the knowledge that you could mess up and others will notice it. I should know, I've performed on stage, and still, I went out and did my best because I had prepared to perform. If I made a mistake, I learned from it and knew that my next performance was a chance to fix it and help my techniques get better. You have everything you need to succeed, just get out in the spotlight so that you can show the world that too. Waiting in the wings will not help you live a fuller and more passionate life.

Some other people that I've spoken to regarding their stage are more private with their passions. They may not want to make a career out of the things that they love, but they still want to continue with their craft because they love it. Still, I tell them that they need to get out onto their stage and show their audience. For these men and women, that audience ends up being themselves. Some people remain focused on a critique they received when they were younger and use that as the catalyst to not pursue their passions as they age. For these people, they don't need to prove anything to anyone else that they love what they love; they have to prove it to themselves. When my self esteem was at its lowest point and I thought to start dancing again, I tried to make excuses for myself to not attempt it. Dancing was something that I loved, but I didn't think that bringing it back into my life would solve the uncertainty and identity issues that I was having. Still, I took a leap and worked through those familiar stretches and exercises and realized that I had nothing to be worried about; my passion was exactly what I needed.

At the time, I needed to just show myself and my family that dancing needed to be a part of my life, but as my passion grew, I realized that I wanted to show the world what I could do with my skills. For many people, they end up sticking to the former scenario and are content with not moving to the latter. That's more than okay; if you're doing something that makes you uncomfortable, then you're not passionate about it and you shouldn't focus any more of your energy on it. Learning what your limits are with your passion as you pursue it is just another way of showing your appreciation towards it.

Whether it's writing poems to your lover or rediscovering your love of dance, don't let the opportunity to showcase your passion pass you by. Get out of the wings and onto your stage; I promise that your performance will be spectacular.

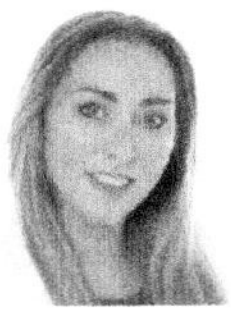

About Rachel Withers

Rachel Withers helps people around the world make mindset, lifestyle and business changes needed to achieve their dreams.

As a business strategist, serial entrepreneur, and public speaker, Rachel applies her experience to coach clients towards personal empowerment and thriving careers. She is the founder of the successful fitness concept BalletBeFit, director of a successful property company, and founder and CEO of business training academy 'Business Growth Hub'.

After founding the successful fitness concept BalletBeFit, Rachel has used her experience to encourage others. Through her courses, Rachel teaches personal development, mindset, wealth mastery, and business development to help each client gain control of their health, well-being, career, and finances. As a public speaker, she captivates audiences around the world with tried and tested strategies for empowerment and growth. Rachel supports people as they build a sense of confidence and learn to apply it within their private and public lives.

Rachel is an Amazon #1 bestselling author, with her book Become a FITPreneur, and has co-authored with the world's leading entrepreneurs and professionals including Jack Canfield to reveal their success secrets, with the best seller 'Success' book. Rachel is a former dancer, who trained with the Royal Ballet, and holds a Bachelor of Performance Arts from Leeds University. She has studied and worked with numerous notable dancers.

When Rachel's dance career ended and she became a mum, her self-esteem took a hit. She realized she needed to make a change for both herself and her family. By transforming her mindset, she used her dance background to develop her ballet-based fitness method BalletBeFit. This mental shift allowed her to surpass career and fitness goals, inspire women to build businesses, and teach her strategies to students worldwide.

On her path to success, Rachel has worked with incredible mentors such as Pat Mesiti and Bob Proctor. She continues harnessing the insights she learned along the way by creating dynamic content for her followers. She hosts the monthly series Mindset Matters on the Success Channel, which has top speakers such as Brian Tracy, Jack Canfield, and Nick Nanton, and uses her experiences and personal development as a way to connect with audiences at her inspirational public speaking engagements. Rachel has been featured on ABC, NBC, CBS and Fox affiliates around the country as a guest of Hollywood live.

Rachel believes we all have what it takes to live the life we deserve. She uses the lessons of her journey to deliver quick results, help her clients discover how to pursue their passion, gain their personal power, and surpass their visions of success and how to implement proven marketing and business strategies. Through Rachel's resources, people learn how to accelerate their progress and self-worth through the power of transforming their mindset combined with entrepreneurship.

Connect with Rachel at:

- info@rachelwithershq.co.uk
- www.rachelwithershq.co.uk
- www.twitter.com/rachelwitherhq
- www.facebook.com/rachelwithershq
- www.instagram.com/rachelwithershq
- www.youtube.com/c/RachelWithersHQ

It's Never Too Late

By Kellie-Anne Fox

As the stage lights hit me, I knew in that very moment I had never ever felt anything more thrilling. It was something I had never felt before. The sound of the audience's applause echoed around the school hall, the burning heat of the stage lights on my face, and my parents and my sister's faces smiling right back at me. At that very moment my passion for dance was born at the age of eleven.

With the world at my feet and my newly found passion, I began to make my journey into the world of the Performing Arts; attending dance classes, joining the local theatre groups, and attending Saturday Stage School. I had started as a shy, inexperienced pupil and by the age of 16, I was at the front of my class. I had achieved this through determination and hard work, through the burning passion I had started with which only grew.

However, just like many in the dance world at the time, I was faced with the problem that I had started too old. Age eleven was just too old and I was told I was lacking in ballet training for me to progress to the next level of professional training. This was the point when my self doubt started. When you are consistently told something, you begin to believe that you are not capable, you are not worthy, and this is the case for many of us. At this point, I had convinced myself that I had indeed started too late and resolved my thinking into becoming a teacher within the performing arts. My studies continued through college and University where I had a Bachelor's Degree in Drama, Theatre & Performance Studies. I continued to work and progressed as a student teacher with my local dance school and the IDTA (International Dance Teachers Association).

With dance comes the stigma of age - are you too old to dance? At what age are we really too old to dance – are we really defined by what society says? How do we overcome this? I had conformed to society; I was too old to dance and succeed, so my passion for dance was extinguished just like a flame from a fire.

As I made my way through the next ten years of my life, I was very lost. I didn't have any interests and I drifted from job to job with no real ambition, if I am honest. All I had known was dance; dance had been my life even though I was always told that I started too late and that I was too old I had been completely defined by society. Not only was I lost, but I never even realized that I had started to lose myself at this point. Who was I? Who had I become? I had always believed that my life must have some purpose, however, I had yet not found that purpose. I was living from day to day, dictated by society to conform to the normal. I find myself now asking myself what is normal? Why are so many of us conforming to the dictated normal?

At 36 I had my son, Franklyn, and seventeen months later my daughter, Matilda, entered the world. My whole identity as Kellie was lost and replaced with Mummy. When you are mother to two small children so close in age, your life focus is the children. At the time, I didn't realize that, little by little, I was just functioning like a robot – lack of sleep, just life in general, but the children gave me focus even if it was always about them. When Matilda was just seven months old, I then found myself as a single parent which was absolutely devastating – my world had been completely turned upside down, but one thing that got me through was the determination and love that I have for my children to continue to thrive and nurture them the best I could. It was an emotional roller coaster to say the least, but most of all, my confidence was non-existent and I was left feeling very useless. My mind was full of so much self-doubt that as a woman, I was not good enough.

When Matilda was just fourteen months old, I began to notice that she did not seem to be walking properly. Her knees looked swollen and she began waking in the night crying, screaming in pain. After four visits to the GP, I then took Matilda to the A&E at my local hospital as the sleepless nights were just too much, as I knew she seemed to be in some form of pain. The only thing the GP had made me feel was that I was just another neurotic mother. However, as a mother you just know if there is something wrong and after attending the A&E and knee surgery. Matilda was diagnosed with JIA – Juvenile Idiopathic Arthritis.

The next year was extremely difficult for me and my children. We attended many hospital appointments and our whole life was focused on Matilda and her care. The care and support that she needed was very demanding, but somehow, I found the strength to keep going. At times I was so alone in all of this, but the one thing I kept telling myself was to keep going and praying that in time it would get better. I was living in hope; the power of hope and the belief that soon life could be better for us all. You learn to live and adapt and that is exactly what I did. I learned how to adapt our life to live alongside Matilda's condition.

In 2018, Matilda was accepted to take part in a medical trial at Great Ormund Street Hospital. The first year was very hard going; it felt at times as if we lived there. So many appointments and check-ups week in and week out, but finally in July of 2019, Matilda began to show signs of going into what they call remission. The arthritis was still there, but it was dormant and controlled by her medication. Finally, she began to walk again after nearly five months of being unable to walk without excruciating pain. Day by day, I worked with her, getting her stronger and stronger. She started walking then was able to run. We worked on climbing the stairs, even if it still presents a challenge, but I have taught her that with enough self-belief she will be able to do anything and achieve all that she wants. Matilda is only four years old and I have tried to instill the power of positive thinking and self-belief in her. What I didn't realize is that I was instilling those same beliefs in myself.

I recall the first time Matilda was able to hold my hand; she was nearly three years of age and due to the pain and swelling that she had in her wrists, hands, and fingers she had been unable to do this. The feeling that I had when I was eleven, back on that stage, hit me again. All that we had been through, the struggle, the life changes we had all gone through suddenly felt irrelevant. In that very moment she held my hand and I felt her fingers lock over mine.

I truly believe that these challenging and difficult times were the making of my journey as I discovered that I had the strength and power to overcome tough situations. This was the turning point for me; I had always believed that I had a life purpose, but I was still yet to discover what this purpose was.

After a fresh start and relocation to the beautiful countryside of Dorset, life began to get better for us all. I began to feel that I needed more and to truly begin my quest to find my life purpose. After reading a newspaper article on Manifesting, I then began to read into this process and then discovered "The Secret," of which I then began practicing the beliefs every day. I learned to be grateful for what I already had and this new positive energy that I had surrounded myself with began to take form; this is when I discovered BalletBeFit by chance. But was this by chance? I believe that I am now truly in control of my destiny. I am the maker of my future and I truly believe that this was no coincidence my purpose; my life journey was about to truly start.

I began my BalletBeFit Instructor Training, bearing in mind I had left the world of dance over fifteen years ago and had not danced since. I was now in training for the very genre of dance that I had always been told I had started too late. My thoughts of the naysayers during my childhood began to resurface, but this time around, I was not going to conform with society. I was not going to be bullied and pressured. I was going to promote the fact that dance is for everyone. My main mission would state that dance is for everyone, no matter your age, and I wanted to unite people of all ages, I would not discriminate. Dance is for any age or any ability, dance is for everyone.

However, on my journey of self-discovery, I wasn't just able to step back in time. I was no longer the dancer that I used to be, mentally nor physically, and that was at times soul destroying for me; already I was missing the confidence that I had so many years ago, but I knew that somewhere deep inside me it was buried within me. The key to my success would be finding it.

The first few months after enrolling into the course, I could barely bring myself to look at the material through fear. Fear is the worst; stepping into the unknown, fear of failure, fear of not being good enough, I told myself I was too tired and that I would do it tomorrow. Don't ever wait for tomorrow because tomorrow never really comes and you will never move forward.

Finally, two months after I took that leap of faith, I literally found a way to overcome my tiredness. As a single parent of two it is exhausting, and it was hard to find that balance between myself and my children after focusing on them for so long. I became involved with every aspect of the training and took the support that Rachel Withers and her team offered. This then drove me forward, but I was left feeling very overwhelmed at times and still didn't have the confidence I needed. The self-doubt creeped back in, the voices kept ringing in my ears about my age. After all, I was forty one, a single parent desperate to get my career back and to have a career to support my children financially. As a single parent I weighed the burden heavily. This was to be my encore, my final moment; I would take the stage once more and fulfil all my hopes and dreams. I religiously started working a rota of timetabled study hours and practical training once I started. I could not believe the progress that I had made within three months. I was in the best place mentally and physically that I had been for years, finally after a few awful years that were very hard for me, I was re-discovering myself. I finally felt that my flame had been reignited within my soul. It's truly amazing as the more that I progressed within the course, the more my confidence started to grow. The more time that I spent with Rachel Withers, the BalleBeFit Team and the BalletBeFit Family, I began to feel purpose. I could finally see everything coming together and I was just about to start my practical exam that I had scheduled for the week after Christmas 2020. My intentions were to start classes at the beginning of the New Year in 2021; I wasn't going to wait. The time was now, finally my time had come.

The morning of Christmas Eve 2020, my children were so excited. We were dancing around to the sound of Christmas songs, the lights on the tree twinkling, the excitement could be felt in the air. Christmas really is such a wonderful time of the year, a time well spent with family. If you look back on your life, I can guarantee your memories are filled with Christmases filled with joy and fun, memories that will last a lifetime.

I returned from the shop with the children. We had been to buy Santa some cookie mix as we were going to bake Santa some cookies this year, the children had insisted. I checked my phone and noticed that my father had tried to ring me several times. He left a text message with the words "Call me Urgent. "As I walked from my kitchen into the bedroom, fear rose up through my feet, I could feel a chill through my veins and my hands were shaking. The words I heard from my father, nothing in my life would have prepared me for this devastating, heart-breaking news. My sister, Nichole, who was only thirty-four, had passed away in the night. No warning, no illness, she was just gone. The words were so final that even now, to this day, the phone call haunts me. My whole world was pulled from underneath me. My words cannot even justify the heart-breaking devastation of that loss, the sudden death of a loved one. The shock is nothing but unbearable. I was now entering a world of the unknown you always hear about with these tragic stories. You always hear about them happening to other people. Suddenly I was that person; I was in complete shock and had no idea of the true meaning of grief until that point in my life.

The next six months were probably the hardest time of my life, many of them the darkest days I have ever encountered both physically and mentally. The complete feeling of loss and heartbreak controlled me, but most of all I felt isolated from friends and family, due to the effects of the Coronavirus and the many lockdowns that we have all been through. Most days I was struggling to function. At times I just could not face the world, but I knew that I had to somehow pull myself together, continue to follow my dream and push forward with my instructor training – however it really was not as simple as it sounded.

Most days, I was physically drained. I felt so overwhelmed that I had a consistent confidence crisis where I had that little voice in my head telling me I could not achieve anything. My passion for success was still there burning inside me. I just knew if I really tried, I could find that strength, I could rebuild myself once more. It seemed the past few years had bought me so much hardship with one thing and another. When you are faced with one final chance to follow your dreams, you have no choice but to step forward and take that step onto the stage. One of my fondest memories of my sister Nichole was that we danced together for many years as children. I have wonderful memories of our dance classes and the many shows that we performed together at the local theatre. The costumes that we wore, the stage make-up, our hair slicked back in the tightest bun glued with about three tons of hairspray, the fishnet stockings, the jazz hands; I felt that Nichole and I conquered it all. These are the memories that I hold dear to my heart and even as I write these words, tears are rolling down my face, my heart is breaking. I can hear her laughing and remember us trying to practice our pickups in our tap class. The most recent memory of her joking around with me was that she was going to most definitely be my first BalletBeFit pupil.

Suddenly my life journey has become so clear; my mission would be to create my own class that would do just this and this is where BalletBeFit Making Memories Workshop was born. It's a monthly workshop that would allow all ages and all abilities to come together to create a memory that would last a lifetime. With this in mind, I was inspired to push myself forward; whether they were good days, bad days, or completely confusing days, I knew that I had to keep going. I began to structure my days once more, often setting myself goals and tasks and, more importantly, surrounding myself with the help and support I needed to get me through. Some days were easier than others and some days I felt as if I was going nowhere. BalletBeFit Lyrical was inspired by my BalletBeFit training and my passion for Lyrical dance. By combining the two, I felt as though I had put my own stamp on teaching this fitness class. I am wanting to spread the message that dance really is for anyone, no experience is necessary. I really want all ages and all abilities to feel welcome. This is my message, but most of all I want to help people create memories with family and friends and bring the community together for all those who have felt lonely and isolated during the lockdown. Life is too short, but really only you can change that. Even on the darkest of days, you must try to overcome the darkness; for once you step out into the light you can certainly know the difference.

Follow your dreams; it really is never too late. I am living proof of this and have done this through the darkest months of my life. I am finally ready to step on that stage once more and I know that my sister Nichole may not be here with me, but she most certainly is waiting in the wings, watching me dance.

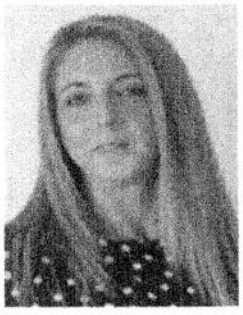

About Kellie-Anne Fox

Kellie-Anne Fox has taken her mission in using dance to create beautiful memories for families to share, her purpose is to make dance accessible for all ages and abilities creating a sense of community to extinguish the feeling of self-doubt and to build confidence and create friendships within her Classes.

Kellie's Classes are for adults, children and she delivers workshops combining the two to create the Making Memories Workshops which is very close to Kellie's heart and her passion has been created from her life journey which drives her forward daily.

As the founder of BalletBeFit Lyrical Kellie uses the technique of BalletBeFit combining this with beautiful lyrical dance movement that comes from her burning passion for dance, the class is to create the ultimate feel good experience with every aspect considered. Dance and Music really do feed the soul and will ignite something deep inside you if you allow it too, but you first must find yourself for then you are able to teach this to others.

The journey for Kellie has been incredible an emotional rollercoaster but one thing that has been consistent is the support that she received from Rachel Withers and her team of which she is and will always be eternally grateful for Rachel's belief in her during one of the hardest years of her life and how if you are believed in that can drive you forward to achieve your life long dreams and ambitions which Kellie is now fulfilling. Kellie's life long passion for dance and fitness began at the age of 11 when she took part in her first school musical production of Joseph & The Amazing Technicolour Dreamcoat. Kellie trained at her local dance school with the examining board IDTA (International Dance Teacher's Association) and then went onto to College to gain a BTEC National Diploma in Dance with distinction and A level Dance,following onto University with a degree in Drama, Theatre & Performance studies.

Kellie truly believes her life journey has bought her to where she is now meant to be, all that she has had to go through has been a lesson even at the most difficult times and days of heartbreak and darkness this has all been to bring Kellie where she is at this present moment in her life, for this is her purpose, this is her destiny but most of all Kellie is now living her life long dreams. Dream It, Wish It, Do It ....

Connect with Kellie at:

- kellie@balletbefit.com

In a World Full Of Copies, Be an Original

By Krystal Longmire

I still remember that last trip we took to the airport as a family unit. I liked airplane rides, so I was excited, but this airport trip felt different. I was about to find out why. Daddy was carrying me, which was normal, but when we got to the airport gate, there was a notable shift in his energy. I have no idea how long we were at the gate, but I remember that my dad was crying. He was holding my head and squeezing me tight and telling me, he loved me. Mommy was standing beside us. She was sad too. Something was off. I could feel it. I think I told my dad that it was going to be okay, and I told him not to cry. An announcement came over the loudspeaker. It was time for us to get on the plane. My dad went to hand me to my mom and my instinct kicked in immediately. Daddy wasn't coming.

I gripped his neck tighter and clasped my hands together. Now, I was crying too. My parents had to pry my fingers apart. My mom tried to take me, but I didn't want to leave daddy behind. Why wasn't he coming? Was this the last time I was going to see him? What was happening? My 5-

year-old mind did not understand. "Daddy, I'm sorry! I'll be good", I shrieked in my mom's ear as I was kicking and shouting. It was that kind of scream that you can hear all the way across the airport; it was blood-curdling and shrill. My mom was holding me tight and telling me it would be okay, and she was crying too. She walked towards the plane to board. My dad told me he would see me soon, and he was still crying, but he wasn't following us. I don't remember that plane ride.

This impactful childhood memory was the beginning of a destructive pattern that had me always trying to fit in with crowds and be like everyone else around me. If it doesn't make sense to you how this one experience could have created a pattern like that, keep reading, and allow me to explain. It wasn't just the divorce that fabricated this mindset; that was just where it originally came from. More accurately, it was also a series of events that happened after that. As I learned later in life, there was a culmination of childhood experiences that drove this pattern deeper into my mind and heart, creating limiting beliefs in my subconscious mind. The truth is, we are all subject to many types of limitations of the mind due to the way we are raised. Our paradigms (habits and beliefs) get created before the age of seven, so it's almost a guarantee that something happened in your childhood too, that created a pattern you might not even be aware of. Your paradigm is where your convicted beliefs come from. When we are children, our minds are like sponges, and we absorb everything. You may have heard this before, and maybe you've even recognized it in your own children as they quickly learn the new things they are taught. I'm not going to go too deep into it here, but I do want to make the point that all humans have a conscious mind (intellectual) and subconscious (emotional) mind. Our conscious mind has the ability to accept or reject new information. The conscious part of our brains can choose not to believe what we experience with any of our five senses. Our subconscious mind, on the other hand, does not have this ability. When it comes to the subconscious mind, everything we experience quite literally gets absorbed.

The reason children are like sponges is because before the age of seven, our conscious mind hasn't developed yet. The amazing thing about this knowledge, is that we all have the power to reprogram our minds. We all have the power to create the reality we desire, but we first must become aware of two things. The first is that the way we think in this very moment was a result of childhood programming that we are likely unaware of. The second is that we are powerful beings with the ability to learn new information and the capacity to overwrite that programming. Until just a few years ago, I didn't know this astonishing truth. After my parents' separation, my time was divided between them. They are from two different cultures, with two different styles of parenting. As I was growing up, I compared myself to those around me and I didn't feel like I fit in on either side of my family. In the beginning, that was primarily because all the cousins I spent the most time with had married parents and I didn't. I was the only one who was sent back and forth. That alone made me different, and I didn't like that feeling. My cousins didn't understand my parents' divorce any more than I did, so as children, our conversations about it made me the odd one out. I remember trying to convince my parents to get back together so I wouldn't be so different. I didn't understand what the problem was. I mean, they should just get back together, right? The mind of a child just truly doesn't get it. During the school year, I lived with my mom in the small town of Wanamaker outside of Indianapolis, Indiana – the heart of the Midwest. When I was with her and her side of the family, I wanted to be like them. I tried to fit in with their personalities.

During the summer, I lived with my dad in a beach town called Luquillo on the island of Puerto Rico. When I was with him and his side of the family, I wanted to be like them. I tried to act and talk like they did. I had lots of fun with both families, and I felt very loved by both parents. In Indiana, we spent long weekends at campgrounds, around campfires, playing in the river, fishing, riding ATVs, going boating and general outdoor living. In Puerto Rico, we went to the beach, neighborhood pools, bike riding, visited water parks and hiked the rainforest. Even with all the fun that was had, the dynamic of each family was so different, and I recognized it even when I didn't understand it. I was only six or seven years old when the transition back and forth started, but I knew that I was living in two different worlds. There was an awkward adjustment period for me when I would arrive in either place, and that lasted my entire adolescence. It was like I had to remember where I was and act accordingly. My parents each had different rules and daily routines, which I'm sure is fairly normal. It was hard to know which way I liked more, which way resonated with "me". Additional changes occurred when I was eight years old, and my dad decided to remarry. When I first found this out, I was slightly devastated. My delusion that my parents would ever get back together was completely destroyed and I was not happy about it. Now, I was never going to be like my cousins. My new stepmom was very nice, and she did everything she could to show me that she loved me just as much as she loved my dad. I could tell that my dad was very happy with her and that he loved her very much, but I felt like she was trying to replace my mom. I was not very welcoming to her in the beginning at all. How could she ruin my master plan?! I did eventually get over my little fit about the whole thing, and thankfully, we have an amazing relationship nowadays. Back in Indiana, my mom never remarried. As a single mom, she worked her butt off to give me everything I wanted. She even ended up getting a second job so she could make ends meet. Raising a child on her own for three quarters of the year could not have been easy. With her second job, she worked weekends and some nights so she was around as much as she could be. Being an only child with no siblings to hang with, I felt lonely all the time. I started finding it difficult to fit in with my friend groups. All of them had siblings. Great. Something else to make me different in elementary school, I was the definition of a tomboy, preferring the company of boys because I got along with them better. I liked wearing baggy clothes, hated brushing my hair, liked to play sports, and I wasn't interested in nail polish or other girly things. I even played with GI Joes, Ninja Turtles, and Matchbox Cars. I also had dark facial hair due to my Puerto Rican heritage, making me feel 'boyish'. The boys let me hang with them, but I didn't fit in all the way, because I was still a girl. So, there I was. Different again. Just like with my cousins, I really wanted to be liked and accepted. I thought maybe I should stop hanging out with the boys so much. Other girls even thought I was weird because I didn't play with them. Any girls that I did hang with were tomboys like me. When it was time for middle school to start, I was so nervous. It was a new school. I had been going to the same school for the last six years with the same group of kids. Now, I was going to be going to a much bigger school that had students from six elementary schools in the township, and that was terrifying.

Somehow, I began befriending the "popular" girls in sixth grade. They were nice enough, but they wore makeup and they dressed differently, and I honestly wasn't sure why they were friends with me. Shortly after my sixth-grade year began, I was pulled into a fight against four eighth-grade girls because I "wasn't pretty enough" to hang out with the friend group I chose. They thought my tom boyishness was weird. I didn't want to be weird. I didn't want to be different. I desperately wanted to fit in and be accepted. I was devastated that my uniqueness had me sticking out like a sore thumb... again. After that, I started wearing tighter clothes and some dresses, so I could "look like a girl". I bought makeup and started waxing my upper lip to avoid getting made fun of for my mustache.

For a while, this worked great. I was "in". That little fight I had gotten into added a bit of a rough exterior for me. I vowed that I would never lose a fight again; that's when my sassy attitude started developing. I didn't realize this at the time, but most of the friends that I gravitated towards were misfits of their own families just like I was. They were also all trying cigarettes, doing sexual things, and experimenting with drugs. I wouldn't say I was a victim of peer pressure because none of them asked me to do what they were doing. However, after feeling for so long like I didn't fit in with my family, it felt so amazing finally having a group of friends that accepted me. Never mind that I changed parts of myself so I could fit in with them.

To continue to be "in" with the "in crowd", I did what they were doing. I vividly remember where I was and who I was with the first time I tried cigarettes and the first time I smoked marijuana. Both made me sick, but I tried to play it off. For each experience, I was staying at friend's houses and begged my mom to let me stay an extra day so she wouldn't find out what I had done. I also felt like I had to figure out how to hide future experiences like these. I assumed since I had done these things once, it would happen again, especially if I was going to keep hanging with this friend group. I had heard the saying, "be your own person", but I never saw anyone practicing it. All my examples seemed like they were following a crowd. Even if that wasn't the case, they all seemed to be LIKE the people around them. No one stood out to me, so I didn't want to stand out either. By the time I got to high school, I was jaded. I had already been in a couple of relationships with not-so-great guys. My first boyfriend in middle school was a year older than me. We both hung out with the same crowds, and we were together every weekend. When he started pressuring me to get intimate with him, I broke up with him. Then, he spread rumors about me. Typical. I had even “dated” a guy who I found out was only “going out with me” as a bet, so that was a fun lesson to learn. Freshman year, I ended up with a guy who was mentally and emotionally abusive. When he put his hands on me, I didn’t leave because he swore he loved me and that he was sorry. I told no one of his transgressions and I stayed way too long because I didn’t want anyone else to leave me. Unfortunately, that was my romantic relationship pattern well into my adulthood, but that’s another story for another time.

The negative attitude that I had developed in middle school after that little fight, got way stronger by this time. I had a huge chip on my shoulder and felt like the world owed me something. I had kept that promise I made to myself. I never lost another fight. I had a lot of fun with my friends, and I was generally happy at school. However, many of my peers were afraid to cross me, both female and male. I walked around with a permanent scowl on my face. I complained about everything and loved finding company with those who were willing to validate my complaints. Everyone knew not to mess with me, and I was proud of that. I also secretly wondered how many of my friends were my real friends and how many were friends with me just because they were afraid not to be. How many of these people just wanted to be on my good side? As crazy as it sounds, I went through my entire high school career like this. At least I was popular now, right? When college began, most of my friends and I all went our separate ways. I was working a part-time job and was going to be attending a full-time schedule of classes. I had a few remaining friends from high school as well as some co-workers, but I didn't have the energy to go through the whole fitting in process by then. I went to class, went to work, and went home, without bothering to get to know any of the people in my classes. I hadn't dropped my rough exterior one bit. My negative mindset and belief that the world owed me something began creating a victim mentality. I was in my early twenties, and my finances were struggling. I blamed these struggles on my circumstances and on other people. In my fourth year of college, I was feeling a bit lost. I had my started college career with a major in the pre-veterinary science field. My grades were fantastic, but no one had told me I was going to have to attend college for twelve years. So, two and a half years in, I changed my major to accounting. I quickly encountered the most boring classes on earth, so I had to get out of that field immediately.

My original minor was Spanish, so I finally changed my major to that instead, even though I had no clue what I planned to do with my degree. I just wanted to graduate. Around that time, through a co-worker, I found West Coast Swing dancing. There was a club that was part of the school, and I began attending regularly. After a few short months, I began dancing competitively. Dancing made me feel alive. Even though my finances were in trouble, I racked up more debt on my credit cards in order to attend the competitions. The dance world I found myself in was a completely different world. I found a lot of new friendships in this world, but I secretly pondered if they were genuine because they sometimes felt superficial. After all these years, I was still wondering if I fit in with this new group of people. Also, even though I progressed in my skill level on the dance floor, I looked around and compared myself to my peers and I always felt like I wasn't good enough. The only way to 'level up' in West Coast Swing is to place in the top five at dance competitions and earn points.

I became obsessed with leveling up because I felt like the more I advanced, the more I would be accepted. I had a great group of friends, but I still really felt like I didn't fit in. My fear of not being good enough shone through on the dance floor, so even though I had advanced my skill level, my confidence and command presence was rarely there, and it prevented me from getting recognized. The people around me were advancing left and right, and I started to lose the love for the dance a bit because I had been stuck at one level for so long. I still danced competitively for years, but the desire to fit in with the crowd hindered me greatly in my overall enjoyment and results on the competitive floor. Fast-forward seven years. I was no longer in college, but I had no degree. I had quit school when I changed jobs. I went from working part time to full time and the schedule demands were overwhelming. Now in the fitness industry, I was working as an Assistant General Manager. Drowning in debt was an understatement. I was overweight and had intense anxiety that often manifested as anxiety attacks, some of which that were debilitating. Having experimented with cannabis back in middle school, I now used it to manage my anxiety symptoms. I had decided that it was impossible to fit in with the crowd, so I completely stopped trying. My negative attitude was out of control by this point. As the 'boss' at my place of business, I used intimidation to gain respect from my staff. Most of them were actually afraid of me, because if anyone got on my bad side, I would not hesitate to pop off. I had a few close friends, but these were also the people I complained about my life and judged others with. I had been through five failed relationships over the past seventeen years, always with less than two weeks in between relationships. I had been hurt so much that I was certain all men were awful, evil creatures who would eventually cheat on me or put me through some kind of abuse.

I had experienced it all, whether that be mental, emotional, or physical pain, and I didn't want to do it anymore. I didn't trust anyone, and I was done putting myself in situations where someone could hurt me. Since I was certain that men could not be trusted, I finally chose to remain single for over a year. I had never done that before. I had never just been on my own by choice. I had a deep need to be accepted and liked. From the very first time I began "dating", I had never been without a relationship for any significant amount of time. I think I felt like if I had a man, I wasn't alone. If someone chose to be with me, that must have meant they accepted me, right? If at least one person accepted me, I didn't have to look for someone else to fit in with. This was such a relief because I had been trying to fit in with people my whole life, but to no avail. I think it gave me a certain kind of comfort to be in a relationship. It somehow didn't matter to me that the people I was selecting as my significant others weren't treating me like I was actually a significant part of their lives; they didn't love me the way I deserved to be loved. Sadly, I had been through so many toxic relationships, I started believing that I didn't deserve to be loved any better than I had been up to that point. Until I chose to separate myself from this dependency on another person, I didn't realize that I was choosing to be in relationships for all the wrong reasons. I didn't recognize how important it was to love myself and be happy on my own before trying to create happiness with someone else.

During this year of alone time, I decided that it was time for me to do the things that I enjoyed instead of always saying yes to everyone else's desires. I picked up some books and started studying personal growth and development. I took a long look in the mirror and realized that I was seriously lacking in self-love. Before my intense self-examination, I had been so worried about fitting into everyone else's mold and being loved by significant others and friend groups, I hadn't even considered loving myself first. Former me was trying to be like others and following the crowd. I was trying my hardest to be the person that everyone around me wanted me to be or at least who I thought they wanted me to be. At the time, it was so important to me to fit into what I believed would be acceptable to others, because if I was accepted, that would mean I was enough. I badly wanted to feel loved for being myself, but as I journeyed down this path of self-discovery, I realized that I had completely lost any sense of self at all. Maybe I never had it. I was almost thirty years old; I didn't have a clue who I was, and I had no idea what I wanted. It was no wonder I had developed a victim mentality and always found a way to spew my negative thoughts on people, complaining every chance I got. Before my own self-realization, if someone would have suggested to me that I was struggling with self-love or that I was unhappy, I wouldn't have believed them.

As a matter of fact, I'm certain that no one in my family knew I was going through emotional turmoil. Hell, I didn't even know it. I felt like I was perfectly happy, and to be honest, I was. I'm sure that after reading my description of everything I went through, it may be hard to believe that I was happy during all those experiences, but from my perception at the time, it's true. All the realizations I'm talking about on these pages weren't discovered or assessed by yours truly until after I had been on the path of healing for a few years. When I did finally take some time to examine my life, I knew for the first time that no one was going to save me from myself. Sure, I had been through things in my childhood, adolescence, and early adulthood, but honestly, who hasn't? I wasn't that different from the millions of people in the world that were trying to figure their lives out. How long was I going to blame the outcome of my world on my past circumstances? I realized that there would always be things that would be outside of my control, but I also always have control over how I choose to respond to those things. On this beautiful ride of learning who I was, I found that I enjoyed spending time with myself. I had fun trying new things and educating myself on what lit up my soul. I rekindled my passion for dance, and I started attending regular social dances, but stopped competing. I got into working out and started taking care of my health on a whole new level. I gave myself permission to try yoga, and I absolutely fell in love. I had been wanting to try it for years, but I was afraid I wouldn't be good at it. Much to my surprise, yoga is a practice that is meant to be a personal journey of self-study. No comparisons. How perfect for this particular time period of my life! I felt fantastic after every yoga class, and I wasn't quite sure why. It didn't matter though. The euphoric feeling was enough to keep me coming back for more. The combination of personal growth, learning to love myself, practicing yoga and meditation and truly investing into my future led me towards the beginning of my self-transformation.

I ended up remaining single for over eighteen months. When I least expected it, as I was conducting interviews at the gym I was managing, I ended up hiring the man who is now my husband. We didn't get along at first, but our friendship blossomed as co-workers, and we developed a tentative relationship after knowing each other for a little over six months. I was still learning self-love and letting go of trust issues when our relationship started. Thankfully, he was extremely patient with me as I rewired my subconscious mind and let go of my limiting beliefs. He was also on his own personal journey of growth and elevation, so it was incredible to be able to share that with him. We have now been together for a little over six years and married for almost three years. I'm so grateful that he came into my life when he did. At the beginning of our relationship, we started attending personal growth conferences together. One of the conferences we attended posed a very important question: "what do you want?" I had already been on my self-love and self-transformation journey for a few years at this point, and I had gone a long way towards finding myself. However, I still hadn't discovered the answer to that question. What DID I want? I had no idea. I was still trying to fit the mold a bit, without realizing it.

My husband wasn't telling me how to live my life, but old habits die hard. He had retired me from the gym with an opportunity he found, and I no longer needed to work a regular job, which was incredible. I truly had the luxury of doing anything I wanted, but I wanted to please him and be a good wife, so I had subconsciously begun following the same path he was on. Honestly, I did this because I thought it was what he wanted me to do (which wasn't true by the way). At this conference, where the man on the stage was asking everyone in the room what they wanted, I learned about the limiting beliefs I mentioned towards the beginning of this chapter. I did an exercise where I poured everything that I ACTUALLY wanted onto a sheet of paper. The first three things I wrote down were dance, yoga, and clean the oceans. However, because of my limiting beliefs, I immediately shut myself down on all three of these desires. I didn't think I was good enough to be a dancer, I thought all yoga teachers were broke and I had no idea where to start with cleaning the oceans. Luckily, I learned that I was placing these limitations on myself; they weren't real, which meant that I could let them go. Nothing was stopping me, but me. When I looked inside myself, I discovered that I actually have a unique gift for helping other people. I understood that I didn't go through my own unique struggles for no reason.

I went through them so I could overcome them. I learned all the things I have learned on my journey so that I could turn around and teach others all the amazing lessons I have acquired. What I wanted was to create an online business that I could use to help women and men let go of their limiting beliefs, learn to love themselves and discover the unique power that lies within each and every one of them too. While I was still at the conference, I registered to get certified in yoga. Shortly after I received my two 200-hour certification, I also got certified in meditation, chakra healing, subtle anatomy, and reiki healing.

I found an amazing mentor who helped me build my online business from scratch. I had no prior knowledge on how to do this, so I was blessed to find her. I became a holistic healer and mindset coach and launched my own wellness business where I help people learn to heal themselves from the inside out. I have an 8-week program, monthly membership, and I offer one on one sessions. I also sell essential oils blends and medical grade water, so I have multiple ways to help people heal in the holistic space. Serving others in this way has been so incredibly fulfilling. I would have never made it to this chapter in my life if I was still stuck trying to fit in with others. As a matter of fact, as I was building my business, my progress slowed a couple of times as I worried how successful I could be if I was doing something that no one else was doing. I recognized this as limiting a belief and pushed past it. This is exactly what I am meant to be doing. I'm not like anyone else and I don't fit into anyone else's mold. I finally chose to follow a path that felt authentic to my heart and soul, and I have helped thousands of people change their lives for the better. My uniqueness is my superpower. Being my authentic self is exactly what makes my light shine so bright, and the same is true for you. Don't worry if you don't fit in. Embrace the beauty of it.

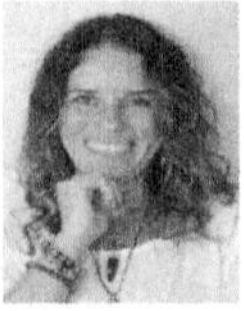

About Krystal Longmire

Krystal Longmire helps people let go of their limiting beliefs, elevate their mindset, release past traumas, and learn to love themselves. This enables people to believe in their own capabilities and create the life they truly desire.

As a holistic healer, natural health aficionado, and mindset coach, Krystal applies her expertise to coach and lead clients towards self-empowerment, healthy lifestyles, and true happiness in every sense of the word. She is the founder and CEO of Krystal Longmire Wellness, the creator of the successful empowerment program Awaken your Inner Power, a leading authority in superior hydration, a specialist in chemical-free living, and your favorite aromatherapy guru.

After creating her flagship program Awaken your Inner Power, Krystal has used her own experience and growth to impact even more lives. Through her courses and one on one coaching, Krystal teaches her clients mindset growth, personal development, yoga principles, nutrition consciousness, and other holistic healing methods to help each client gain control of their own personal wellness; to thrive in mind, body, spirit, and emotions.

Krystal holds certifications in Yoga, Primordial Sound Meditation, Chakra Healing, Yoga Nidra, Subtle Anatomy, and Reiki Energy Healing. As a holistic healer, she guides people all over the world to let go of the self-imposed limitations that are keeping them stuck in a life that doesn't serve them. Krystal supports people as they build their inner confidence and step into their true power, helping them learn to apply their growth in all aspects of their public and private lives.

Krystal formerly worked in the fitness industry for ten years and holds a Bachelor of Arts in Spanish from Indiana University. She is bilingual and proficient in the art of translation. She has helped break communication barriers in many different industries over the years. When Krystal abruptly left the fitness industry due to her husband's change of career and location, she was completely lost. She had lost her excitement for her field over time, and realized she needed to find her passion to be truly happy. She elevated her mindset, let go of limiting beliefs, and created her first program, Awaken your Inner Power. This mental shift allowed her to go after and achieve her goals, inspire men and women to be their authentic selves in their personal and professional lives, and share her wisdom with mentees everywhere.

On her path to success, Krystal has worked with incredible mentors such as Bob Proctor, Tony Robbins, and Deepak Chopra. She is constantly continuing her own growth and passing down her insights through empowering content creation for her followers. Krystal believes we were all meant to live life that dreams were made of. She uses her own trials and tribulations, as well as her experience helping others to help her clients learn to love themselves, believe in their own power, let go of limiting beliefs, and create the lives they truly desire. Through Krystal's resources, her clients elevate their mindset, heal their past traumas, and transform into the best and happiest version of themselves.

Connect with Krystal at:

- www.krystalsworld.com
- Healingwithkrystal1@gmail.com
- https://www.instagram.com/healingwithkrystal
- https://www.facebook.com/healingwithkrystal

A Whole Waterfall

By Deborah Ruddy

I was sitting looking at the red light, waiting for it to change to green and for the traffic to move again when BANG!!

My life changed at that moment. I could hear the crunching sound of the metal and I could feel my body forced forward at the same time, shoved back into the seat as the airbag hit my sternum and the seat belt snapped back to hold me in my seat. Those few seconds seemed to last forever. I could hear myself moaning and then heard someone shouting.

I had been rear-ended at full force. I wanted to get out of the car to see the damage, but the gentleman who came to my aid would not let me. I was still in my seat, the force of the airbag had winded me, and he wanted to make sure I didn't hurt myself more. My concern was weirdly for my car and not myself; I had only bought it two weeks prior, and it was my pride and joy. The man stayed with me to wait for an ambulance. He was so very kind, and I was so very sore. It wasn't until I was loaded into the ambulance that the heaviness of what exactly happened to me hit. I didn't realise it at the time, but the accident was my first step on a wonderful journey into holistic wellness.

Fast forward ten months later: I was back in the hospital for a similar situation. There was repeated injury to my spine and neck. The doctor told me that all of the soft tissue in those areas were severely damaged. There was a road to recovery that involved plenty of Physiotherapy but one that I tried to face as positively as I could.

One day, as I sat feeling sorry for myself, I remembered the words from one of the first responders on the scene of my first accident. When I was in the ambulance, being rushed to the hospital he said, "I have been to accidents with less damage and people don't walk away."

Those words stuck with me. There I was, two accidents down that had both cars I drove totaled in the process, but I had been lucky enough to walk away. Yes, I was injured, but I was alive and pretty much in one piece. There was pain, but it could have been so much worse. I knew I needed to focus on that positive mindset, in order to assist with my recovery.

Physiotherapists became my friends and work became my enemy. I was working fifteen-hour days in a high-powered job with lots of stress that did not work for the body I now had. Either I tried to find something I could do outside of the office before or after my shift to help alleviate the pain and tension my body was feeling. I first attempted to try going to the pool before work, doing some water exercises that would take the pressure off, of my neck and back, but it was difficult to fit in around my work commute and work schedule. I knew I needed an alternative.

One of my therapists suggested I try yoga. It was something I was able to find multiple classes for and I decided to commit to a six-week program. The studio was near my workplace, so I knew I would not miss it. Even if I needed to schedule myself for a class during my work hours, I'd be able to get over to the class without issue, which didn't leave me any excuses not to go.

Sitting in my first yoga class, a part of me wished that I had done some research on it. I had committed to six weeks of a class that I didn't know the first thing about. The recommendation was one of many I'd received over the few months after my second accident and I hoped that yoga would be able to do something for my pain. My back was feeling particularly bad, and I was dreading whatever exercises that the instructor would have me attempt.

Without even knowing it, this was the first true step on my road to recovery, not just physically, but mentally as well. That road led not only to healing, but also to the revelation of my inner self and allowing a 'new' me to shine after being hidden away for so long. I didn't realise just how much of myself I had closed off when I was growing up. I know that there are probably a few people reading this book and being surprised to know that about me, but it was something I didn't even realise until I was older. I had a belief that the people I surrounded myself with were more athletic, prettier, more confident, more intelligent, or were just plain better at things than I was. My insecurities and lack of confidence caused me to shelter myself and I allowed myself to be overshadowed by my comparisons to everyone else.

I look back on that time without regret, since I know that learning to accept the decisions, I made in the past has helped me to understand that there was already a set path out for me to get me to where I am now. My journey with yoga assisted in helping me to reflect on my past and learn more from the decisions that I made. Yoga gave me a conduit, in order for me to look after my body, mind, and spirit in tandem. The six-week yoga course wasn't the class for me, but I found an instructor that I just clicked with. I met her while speaking at a conference and I found that I connected with her on a level that I wasn't fully aware of. I was still in pain from my injuries but slowly and gently I found my road to recovery through her teachings and support.

While I was working through my classes, I read a book called *Say Yes to Life by Dr Linda Finnegan and Christy Kenneally*. The first chapter in this book is "Recognize your Resilience" and one of the lines spoke to me: "At certain time in our lives we can reach the depths of our own despair. During these emotional winters, our future can appear bleak, and our hope larder can seem terribly bare. But is it really bare?" After all of my experience, I can answer that question with a resounding 'no'; you have resources within you to reach for, you just have to dig deep enough to find yourself. You need to allow the crazy world to melt away and let yourself shine so that you no longer have to wait in the wings for your turn. Give yourself the benefit that you've got more in you than you think, and you'll be amazed by what you discover.

Start to listen to the Inner Child

Our inner child dreams big, has a wild imagination, and believes that everything is possible. When do we stop listening to that voice? Tuning into the voice of our inner child is never more important than when we become adults. Don't stifle the child within; this can be where real innovation happens and how we can find our true happiness. Remember nothing is beyond our reach, we are merely blocked by our own limitations.

Begin to get to know yourself

Take some time and get to know yourself. I'm sure that you hear that a lot from self-help books and guided meditation, but there's not a lot of explanation out there on just how to know yourself. From my experiences, there are a few ways to do this. There are the usual probing questions that you can ask yourself and write those answers in a journal. Journaling helps to get your unedited thoughts down on paper for you to reflect on, which helps you get a sense of what your state of mind is like on certain days and at certain times. Meditation also provides a way for you to focus on aspects of yourself and take time to reflect on those aspects. I found that a mixture of the two helped me to get in touch with who I really am, but it's important to understand that this doesn't happen overnight. I was familiar with self-reflection from a retreat I had gone on when I was a fifth year. I went to a Catholic secondary school and the retreat was described to us in a way that would have us out of school, but still learning about our religion. I was a teenager, so I was just happy to have a few hours out of school. We had group sessions at the retreat and one of them, in particular stood out to me; it focused on our futures and what we were planning to do after we completed secondary school.

The questions were presented bluntly: what kind of career are you thinking about, where do you see yourself in five years? I was one of the few students that was able to answer the latter question and I told the person leading our group that I saw myself in a job that would have me in a nice car and let me take holidays abroad. At the time, not many people took holidays out of the country, but I wanted to be able to get the chance to. My peers all spoke about their plans for going to a good college and getting their master's or PHD, I wasn't even thinking about having more schooling. I remember feeling out of the loop for the rest of the session, since the leader decided to focus on speaking about what college would be like and what kind of work would be expected. After the retreat, I allowed myself to think about what sort of things I liked that would get me into a career that I'd enjoy. I liked sports and participated in cross country running and played basketball with the school team. I began thinking about what kind of career would have me in a setting where I would provide services related to fitness, but my teachers noticed how well I succeeded in maths, and they encouraged me to investigate something related to business or accounting. I let other people talk me out of something I was truly interested in and a part of me wonders what my life would have been like if I had pursued my fitness career as soon as I left school. Still, deep down, I know I was destined to be on this road, no matter what bends or wrong turns I took along the way. My life is no less full because it took me years to get back to my passion.

Here are some probing questions you can ask yourself and journal on. Remember to be open and honest; your answers are for your eyes only and can serve as tools of reflection as well as providing guidance about your truth:

When you smile, what brings that smile to your face? List as many things as you can think of. When you are finished, see how many are similar.

- What do you love to do even if you are tired?
- What is your biggest fear?
- We all have them, don't ever dismiss them, so write down what you're truly afraid of.
- What is your biggest dream? It does not have to be anything that actually exists, it can be a complete fantasy.
- Who in the world do you admire, what is their best quality?
- Would you stay in an unhappy relationship? That relationship does not have to be a partner (boyfriend / girlfriend, husband / wife) it can be someone like a parent, brother, sister, etc. This question might be a bit difficult to answer, but the reflection is worth it.
- What would you most fear about finishing an unhappy relationship?
- What is your biggest achievement to date?

- What is your relationship with your parents / family like?
- What qualities would your friends say you have?
- How do you feel about failure?
- What is your relationship with money like?
- Who do you least like to spend time with?

Begin to surround yourself with like-minded people

Think about the people you surround yourself with. Are they there to fully support you in everything you do or are there some who don't care if you succeed? This can be harder than you think to spot. When you start on your journey through life, you think everyone has your back and will want you to succeed; however, you may notice just an odd remark here or there that can make you doubt yourself. This does not necessarily make these people bad, but it is not their journey.

The doubts or fears that they bring up are more to do with them and their doubts and fears than with yours. These doubts can really keep you in the wings and prevent you from stepping out into the limelight that you so deserve. When you are on your journey in life, you will begin to find your tribe, the like-minded people and the ones who support you. Don't attempt to compare yourself to anyone else that is in the same business as you; be content with who you are and be confident within your abilities. Allow yourself to shine. I remember when I started out, I taught for a long time to just three people. However, my students were loyal and are still my clients today. Don't lose faith, build a foundation, and then grow it.

Speak to yourself as if you were speaking to your best Friend

Be mindful of the language you use when you speak to yourself. Quite often, we can speak very negatively towards ourselves; however, it is so important to change that mindset.

You would never tell your best friend, "You are stupid, you don't know what you are doing. Who would want to learn from you?" These damaging words of self-obliteration need to stop. We may not believe that we're the greatest person in the world, it is vital that we talk ourselves up and believe in ourselves more. Doing the work that you want to do will give you confidence. Knowing that you have completed all that you need to be an expert in your field gives you a strength of mind that you are able to achieve your dream. I remember my very first class I had when I was just beginning to teach. I was nervous and I am sure I messed up while speaking, but I took the time to acknowledge any error I made, and it only showed I was human and set the class at ease. I was able to get through it slowly, but, more importantly, safely. When you are an instructor, you hold a place on a pedestal for your students as the person they look to in order to complete their lesson. From your point of view, you are ensuring that the environment is safe, that the students feel comfortable, that you are able to set everyone at ease and be inclusive, that you can provide adaptations if necessary, and that you're providing a space where students can have fun and enjoy what they are doing. While health and wellness can be serious and you want to provide the best for your students, it is okay to have some levity in a class, as it settles the minds of the students and allows them time to enjoy their class but at the same time feel like they have worked out.

So, remember when speaking to yourself, speak as if you were talking to your best friend. Build yourself up with affirmations of, "You have got this, you will be fine. The students will love your classes; they are here for you and what a wealth of knowledge you have to give."

Remember Self-Care

Self-care was the main reason that started my journey to be an instructor in the wellness industry. It's also been the most important factor in keeping me where I need to be. We need to challenge ourselves and push ourselves out of our comfort zone in order to reach our goals but listening to our bodies and minds and knowing when to take a break is vital. There is a saying: "You cannot pour from an empty cup." It's a bit self-explanatory, but let's dive deeper into what is actually being said. If there is nothing in a cup, then all you are pouring is nothing, right? The same goes for the human body and mind; if you don't look after it, you won't be able to give anything to those around us who we love and care for. If you're feeling empty, then you need to take care of yourself in order to become full again.

Some may say that self-care is selfish, but, personally, I think it is selfless. After my accidents, if I had not listened to my body and looked after it, I don't know where I'd be now. If I'd never listened to the physiotherapists and completed the relevant programs, I needed to assist in recovering the strength and stability in my body, there's a likely chance that I wouldn't be able to move. Even though I've recovered somewhat, I still continue to listen and know what my limits are. It can be frustrating to put limits on yourself, especially after I've just explained about how you can do anything, but if it means that you won't be happy and healthy when you reach your goal, then what's the point?

When I began my instruction in Anti-Gravity Aerial Yoga, it did wonders for my spine and flexibility. I continued my training and became a Suspension Fitness Anti-Gravity Aerial Yoga and Restorative Anti-Gravity Aerial Yoga instructor, the latter becoming my niche. I loved how the body could assist in healing itself and, with the assistance of the hammock, could build on that healing. I love that I'm able to assist others in their healing as well. When I instruct my classes, I try to instruct from a place of empathy. I know first-hand how hard it can be to touch your toes; after my accident, I couldn't even bend over to touch my knees. I have continued my training as a 500 RYS Yoga Instructor and a BalletBeFit Instructor and all these disciplines combined not only complement one another but assist in gaining strength and stability in your body as well as improved flexibility. I think when you look at restoring the body you can find not only a cup to pour from, but a whole waterfall.

I am so grateful for the journey I have been on, as it has allowed me to step out of the wings and into centre stage.

I may not be totally comfortable with the spotlight on me, but I can certainly cope with the glow, I guess we are all a work in progress. I will leave you with this thought from Lou Holtz:

"Ability is what you are capable of doing. Motivation determines what you do. Attitude determines how well you do it."

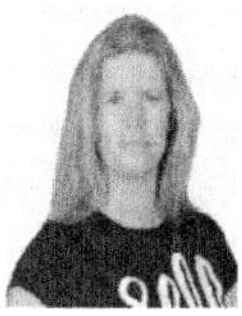

About Deborah Ruddy

Deborah Ruddy is a qualified Anti-Gravity Aerial Yoga instructor, which was her first step into the fitness industry, she continued as a student of yoga and meditation where she decided to take it a step further and explore the gift of yoga. She is now a RYT 500hr Yoga Alliance qualified Yoga Instructor who is passionate about finding a balance between body, mind, and spirit.

She created her brand Lila Fitness, "Lila" a Sanskrit word meaning Devine Play. Deborah believes that life can be stressful enough so when you arrive at one of her classes that you can find levity and fun while rebuilding strength and flexibility back into the body and through this restorative body you will build a restorative mind and spirit.

Deborah is aware of her own flexibility and her own body limitations but embraces them and brings that empathy through to her yoga classes. Through her fitness business she has added on classes such as mediation and BalletBeFit which fit with her ethos of rebuilding and restoring the body and mind. Deborah mentors on VTSOY 200hr Teacher Training, which she has had first-hand experience of as this was the school of yoga that she came through. She helps to bring new students through their journey to yoga and guides them on their new path. Deborah formerly worked in a very corporate environment in both Finance and Retail before she entered the fitness world, so she understands a busy and stressful working life. Deborah wants to continue to add wellness strategies to her business and continues with her personal development to offer new elements as she grows her business. So, Deborah and Lila Fitness will bring a balance to you and your Mind, Body, and Spirit to re-charge your life so that you build yourself the best life.

Connect with Deborah at:

- www.lilafitnessire.com
- Instagram: @lilafitnessire
- Facebook: @Lilafitness1
- lilafitnessire@gmail.com

It's Time To Go Dance

By Judy Wong

Prologue
When my friend Rachel Withers asked me to write this chapter for her book, I was deeply moved. Being a late-comer to the self-exploratory art of dance, it has been the most excruciating and rewarding body, mind and soul exercise that I have ever taken on in my years of life on this planet. For you, who is reading this book, do not wonder, do not hesitate, do not sit on the verge of the greatest and most intimate adventure you'll ever have with yourself. Just take that very first step, the rest will follow....

Introduction
"In the end, we only regret the chances we didn't take, relationships we were afraid to have, and the decisions we waited too long to make." Before I dive into how and why I think everyone needs to take up dancing as part of their regular activity, I want you to realize that this is such an amazing journey that I wouldn't trade it for all the material pleasures that we often get caught up in the corporate world.

As I commit pen to paper for this chapter, during the midst of a global pandemic, I can tell you as a matter of fact that we have all accumulated some false beliefs during our time here on earth. I used to be the most insecure and un-confident person when it came to my body. Having an Asian heritage made me prone to stereotypes that left me feeling sub-standard, too fat, too muscular, too big boned, not tall enough, etc., etc, and undesirable. So much so that I would dismiss the very thought of being in front of the camera, avoid photos at most gatherings, and be the first one to bolt for the door at the thought of being in the limelight.

My stage fright was so debilitating that just the thought of being in front of people and doing more than reading off power point slides (when conducting training in the corporate world) would make my hands shake, my stomach churn and make me want to vomit! Yet, somehow I learned through this unravelling process called dancing to undress all the garbage that covered my soul. I learned to dress in costumes that I never imagined possible for my body type (i.e. Very little fabric), get on that dance floor and flaunt it like my life depended on it!

Our bodies are truly our temple. We are only given one shot in the bodies that we're given and it's a shorter journey than you think. So if you've been "thinking about it" it's time to stop thinking, get off that couch and get moving!

In The Beginning

I was 35, a mother of a toddler, in between jobs as a highly paid executive working for a Wall Street corporation in Hong Kong, the hub of Asian markets (excluding Japan), and I was married to my high school sweetheart. Nothing on the surface could have been more perfect to the eye of the beholder. I had always been quite disciplined about maintaining my health and body, I had always been convinced that I wanted to stick around on the planet a little longer. Life as a full time mom was really getting to me. I was miserable and sad. I was immensely frustrated with my life and the so-called lifestyle that everyone supposedly dreamed about. I thought to myself, "People wrote fairy tales about this type of life?! DAMN ~ Either I am not fairy tale material, or somebody's been trying to deceive all of woman kind!" My Master's degree had gone to waste, as I sat there in my living room thinking about what to cook for dinner - carrots? Beef? "How the hell do I know what he wants to eat?" My marriage was highly dissatisfying to say the least. I felt resentful for the life I had chosen.

"Ding!" The WhatsApp message prompt on my phone got my attention. A new friend whom I had made at a dinner gathering messaged me and asked if I wanted to go dance with her next week. I felt a glimpse of excitement followed by a moment of doubt.

Dance? What did she mean "dance"? Like bite a rose and wiggle my ass? (It's called Tango by the way -- I later learned the name of this style of dancing.) She later explained that it was great cardio, and that the doctor's had ordered her mother who was over the age of 70 to get some cardio exercise each week and asked if I wanted to accompany her. To say that I was a bit reluctant was an understatement. I was happy with just practicing yoga asanas, and I am usually a great sport, but anything that involves me moving with grannies was really a bit too much for me. I wasn't prepared to humiliate myself. I was wondering why I didn't opt for doing tai-chi in the park instead.

"When was the last time I *truly* danced?" I asked myself. Flashback to night clubs on King Street in Toronto during my high school & college years, fake IDs, bouncer friends who would let me in the door while under-age, eating Vietnamese pho noodles at four am on Spadina Avenue, scarfing down street-vendor polish sausage hotdogs in minus twenty-five degree Celsius (as was the typical Canadian winter), and hanging with the crew. The crew were my tightest friends at the time, most of my friends being male, it always felt safe to go clubbing with them. I always knew someone would have my back in case some horny guy couldn't keep his hands off me (of course there's nothing wrong with attracting a little attention...Why else would we go clubbing?!). Amongst these male friends, there was a tight group of four who called themselves the 4-horsemen who apparently thought they brought the apocalypse to the night clubs. The Asian girls would be gagaing in their presence, they would bust out their kung-fu moves and move to the rhythm of the music, and by the end of the night they would then compare who got the most phone numbers in the car on the way home (if they all made it back into the car).

I recalled the thumping sound of the base being so loud that I felt my whole body shake. I remember the DJs mixing up tunes that would make the crowd cheer with excitement. I remembered how my body would naturally wave, my feet would naturally move, and when it was all over, me, the nerdy, responsible big sister occasionally got stuck being a designated driver. With my less-than-awesome driving skills I would drive someone's car in three feet of snow & ice because all my friends were too drunk to ever pass a Breathalyzer test.

Then my mind fast forwarded to high-end lounges by Sydney Harbour Bridge when I worked on assignment in Australia. I may have grooved a bit to the music in my corporate attire during happy hour alongside friends in suits. After that, my mind went blank. "When was the last time I *truly* danced?" I asked myself.

I let out a big sigh of nostalgia. My glory days, before I got married and picked up responsibilities like a kid, a husband who never grew up, a mortgage, an executive job and a whole lot of corporate political bull shit. With a bit of prompting on my friend's part, I agreed to join her. I attended my very first class on nothing more than an apple for breakfast -- BIG mistake! I thought she'd make me sway my hips at the most.

The Journey

I was very in touch with my body, or so I thought. Yoga asanas were a big part of my twenties. I had always been active and I had recently had a child and gone through the both joyous and depressing moments of new-found motherhood.

In that very well-lit studio classroom I learned very quickly that I knew very little about my body. A built, tanned,

South-East Asian instructor walked into the classroom. When the music went off, I started to move to the beat of the music to the best that I could and tried to mimic the instructor in the front of the room.

The class was supposed to last ninety minutes. At the forty-minute mark, I thought I was going to pass out. Having only an apple for breakfast, my blood sugar levels were plummeting and I had sweat so much I was convinced I had just lost two pounds! I actually had to sit on the ledge at the back of the class room and heaved away trying to catch my breath. My legs felt like they were going to cramp, and I had already done some yoga stretches in the morning before I attended class. I stared at the clock on the wall and I do recall thinking, "This is the longest ninety minutes of my life! When is this going to end!" Then I glanced over and within a few feet of me, my friend's mother, over seventy years old was bouncing away, happy and smiling with all sweat dripping all over the floor. I cannot remember if I growled out loud, but inwardly I was definitely growling. I couldn't be worse than a seventy year old, I was half her age! So I dragged my butt back to my spot on that dance floor and started moving. I can no longer recall what I ate after class, but after burning around nine hundred calories, I was convinced having cheesecake was justified.

Graduating From Kindergarten

Fast forward two years of dancing like a maniac, learning how to control my limbs, and realizing my knees were beginning to hurt from all the impact, I decided to "try something different". Feeling good really is addictive. I didn't know what I had done right or wrong, but I knew that my body was beginning to show signs of living a truly aligned life. My physique was more slim and toned, yet I was feeling the impact of prolonged friction on my knees. I knew that if I wanted to continue having so much fun, I needed to "try something different" and minimize the wear and tear on my body. I didn't even really know what "different" meant, I only knew that I had friends who were much bigger than me in size who kept telling me I had to go try something different.

Eventually I stopped questioning and just took their word for it, fully acknowledging that it was related to dancing and that they weren't suddenly asking me to go start rock-climbing or something like that! Deep within the recesses of my mind though, the image of the woman biting a rose with some guy holding her waist flashed into my mind. "Ummm, not me. No thanks. I am married," I thought. If this is what they had in mind, I would totally need to strangle at least two girlfriends.

All my false misconceptions held me back from exploring yet another facet of my existence, until one day someone asked me if I wanted to try jazz. The image of a saxophone popped in my head. That, and an image of Katherine Zeta-Jones performing in Chicago, the Broadway musical. Well, I did learn a little ballet as a child (as most little girls in first world countries do) and so I agreed to try this "jazz-thing". I arrived at that particular studio in Tsim Sha Tsui about fifteen minutes early. It was dark. It had black and yellow walls and low ceilings. Instinctively I thought about my teens and twenties spent clubbing in downtown Toronto.

Clubbing didn't require skill, it required a tight skirt, a low v-neck shirt, a drink with ice that would last all night, and the bobbing of my head to the bass. "I wonder if they're going to turn off the lights? This jazz thing was going to interesting," I thought.

On the hour, enters a tanned, older man (my guess was late forties to fifties), dressed in modern attire. He hooks up the sound system and I noticed everyone taking their places on the dance floor. To say that I was intimidated was an understatement. I actually got through warm ups quite easily because I was flexible, but then came the hard part. This class didn't have many songs. This class had one song and one song only. The purpose of this class was to keep repeating that one song over and over again. I was silently hoping that I would know the music because I was doomed otherwise. Without having anyone formally tell me, I was initiated into the world of choreography. Choreography as the almighty Google Dictionary defines it, "is the sequence of steps and movements to a dance." This is what the professionals do. Me, I was just there to observe and move my limbs. I stood there at the back of the room with my hyper-critical self-judging words, watching the others move to the music and wondering how the heck I was ever going to execute something like that without the instructor at the front of the room for me to follow. "Memorize the steps!" Shouted the instructor from the front of the room. Wow, memorizing the steps? When was the last time I worked my memory in this way? I had no idea. Memorize the sequence? This was going to be harder than playing poker, or mahjong, where I had to remember what cards had been dealt.

"Memorize the steps and flow with the music!" Shouted the instructor. I am no brain surgeon, but I knew that the human mind can only build new neuro-pathways through repetition. With zero experience, I also knew at the time that I would be lucky if I could perform thirty seconds of music without looking like I was imitating Barney the purple dinosaur on a kids show! It turned out to be a very nerve-wracking class of me comparing myself to everyone else. Since then, I have tried many different styles of dancing; heels, chair, contemporary, hip hop, waltz, salsa and even bachata. All of these styles allowed me to explore far beyond the limitations of my body, flexibility and agility. Of course, all of those aspects are important and are useful when learning a new style of dance, but the real purpose behind my learning to dance was far deeper. For me, dancing allowed me to explore a long buried side of my personality, one that I had forgotten even existed. I encountered many amazing choreographers who all have their own unique style, their own story, and through their own life experiences have formulated different ways of teaching and execution. Each piece of music is often chosen for a particular reason, the beat, the lyrics, the mood it creates. The steps are also often carefully considered in accordance with the level of difficulty that students are able to take on. What appears to be easy and natural, is actually all part of a carefully formulated plan on the part of the instructor to help the student achieve progress. In the midst of every class, there was an array of people. Students who were there to truly improve their skills, those who were there only recreationally to enjoy themselves, those who were there to get fit and those who were there to enhance their sensuality. There's one thing that we all agree on, and that is that dancing is liberating. Occasionally there would be a party pooper who would complain about how they didn't enjoy a class, but in all honesty, that was rare. Unless there was an accident, where someone fell, someone got stepped on, someone hurt themselves by pushing themselves too hard, every lesson was an opportunity to go deeper.

The Mirror, The Lessons

When you need to face yourself in the mirror, it's really one of the most petrifying sights. You're forced to look in the mirror to see whether you're actually performing a movement the way that you're supposed to. This also means that you're forced to look at your body and all of its imperfections in the way that you move, the way that you express and the way you try to convey a message to the audience.

As a woman and a relatively new mother, I had to look at the havoc I had done to my body. I had to admit to myself the pain of having loved a man that didn't love me, how I gave my body to bear his child, how my body had been thwarted, stretch-marks and all, how my skin was no longer as tight and taught as when I was in my teens or twenties. I looked at my hips, my thighs, my not-so-perky boobs and asked myself what I had done. Please do not misinterpret my remarks as being ungrateful for having the child that I have. I am immensely grateful each day for God having made me a mother. What I do want to emphasize though, is the pain that came from the constant and daily confrontation that I had with the mirror that forced me to look myself in the eye and ask whether this was the life that I was prepared to live. A life of servitude to societal norms and expectations, or a life of self-love, self-devotion and dignity.

I used to think that dancers are highly skilled athletes. In fact, they are that and a lot more. Dancing, unlike other sports, require more than just the vigorous training of the body, and to a large degree the mind. Dancing requires that the dancer be highly in touch with his or her emotions. It is the one sport where you are not only encouraged to feel, but to express those emotions. This in my opinion has been one of the toughest lessons and the most excruciating lesson. In order to fully execute a piece to the music, we sometimes need to excavate long lost emotions that have been deeply buried in our past. Sometimes, you'll know what a dancer has been through in their life simply by the way that they express themselves to a piece of music.

After living years in an emotionally dissatisfying relationship, which turned into a sour marriage, I decided I really had no idea what it meant to "be sexy", never mind "dance sexy". That was something I learned in jazz class. The combination of instructors taught me the difference between moving my body versus feeling sexy from both a male and female perspective. The two are not the same. You can physically dance the steps and it can appear to have zero sexiness to it. I even recall the first thought I had when I was once asked to open my legs in a straddle and then clip my legs together. I was mortified. "Spread my legs like that and then clip them?! I cannot open my legs like that! I'm a mom!" I later learned that being a mom should mean opening my legs is not rocket science - after all, I must have practiced the act of sex in order to conceive!

The next challenge was that of being in the spotlight. I was just not a person who enjoyed attention. In fact, I dreaded attention. Outside of the office where I made many presentations while relying on power point presentation slides, I didn't enjoy being in front of a camera. I didn't like to wear make-up and I assumed that attention seekers must be highly emotionally bankrupt to demand that people pay attention to them all the time. So many assumptions right? Yes, this is precisely what goes on in the head of a newbie dancer. A whole lot of doubt and worry.

When the chance to enroll in a "showcase" came up, I was too scared to sign up. I had massive performance anxiety. After much pushing and encouragement from two plus-size girl friends, I reluctantly signed-up. I knew the style of dancing would be jazz. What I didn't expect was that there would be costume requirements. I wasn't afraid to show some skin, but I was definitely uncomfortable with the idea of showing skin and dancing supposedly-sexy at the same time! I vividly recall my very first performance on stage to that jazz routine, I was wearing something the resembled a bra/lingere with black pants, a black hat and a black jacket. I was so nervous and scared, that despite the stretching and breathing exercises I did backstage, I was still practically hyper ventilating in the wings, and I went to the bathroom to pee every five minutes before it was our turn to be on-stage. I felt like I had suddenly developed bladder problems just before the show! In the end, I survived the performance. I didn't forget any steps, although the execution was not great, and very fortunately for me and all my fellow peers, I did not vomit everywhere. My jitters persisted until long after the show was over. I could hardly believe I had actually pulled it off! The next thing I knew I wanted to try was contemporary dance.

I learned very quickly that having flexibility was a very basic part of contemporary dance. In fact, in order to do any of the pieces properly, a basic understanding of ballet foot positions was definitely helpful. Contemporary dancers often incorporated some very sophisticated gymnastic jumps in their routines. It was not something I needed to try as an adult, but it was definitely an art form that required more than just memorizing steps and understanding music. It was about a lot more than just the lyrics. Sometimes the pieces would have no lyrics, and you truly had to "feel" into the piece. Those were the routines that really took me to new heights, perhaps not because of the turns, but because of the need to tap into myself.

While all styles of dance intrigued me, short of my love-hate relationship with ballet, contemporary class was always something I wanted to try. Why the love-hate relationship with ballet you may ask? Well, that's simple, as a child in ballet class I was told that I was too chubby that I didn't have the right build and that I didn't have what it would take to go beyond a recreational class. I was told that I was unfocused and distracted others in the class --

whoops, so much for enjoying yourself as a kid ballet was for serious pretty & thin children with serious ambition. It wasn't for chubby Asian girls growing up in the 1980's in Canada,

I wasn't sure what was worse, being Asian and an ethnic minority or being chubby. So, contemporary dance was always something I aspired to try but was too intimidated to start. Perhaps one of the greatest blessings on my dance journey was stumbling into a seasoned contemporary choreographer by the name of Ahmir. She would disapprove of how I labelled her as "seasoned" and "contemporary choreographer", because she's youngish and dances many different styles. How did I meet her? Well, remember that dance studio I mentioned earlier which had a black and yellow walls? Well, it eventually closed its doors. That studio failed at extending its lease negotiations with the landlord and was forced to close. After its closure, I randomly stumbled into another "more reliable" studio. "More reliable" defined as a studio which had a longer reputation in the market. Let's not forget, even dance studios are business ventures. Studio owners face the same pressures as any other bricks and mortar business which relies on providing recurring services to retail customers.

So, one random Saturday afternoon I walked into this "more reliable" studio which operated several locations throughout the city. I looked at the schedule, saw a class labelled as "Sexy Funk" and decided I felt "sexy" enough to try. I was wearing black, "Black is always sexy," I thought. When I walked into her class, it felt like I had crossed the threshold through the closet and into Narnia. Warm-ups alone were unlike any other adult class I had attended! She truly treated all of us grown woman (with some ladies in their 60s) as if we were dancers in our twenties. Warm-ups were intense. Splits, back-bends, bridges, crunches, partner stretches and partner lifts for strength training. Jumps, turns, drills. She called it baby-training. (Meanwhile, half of the class had trouble figuring out their left side from right side, and how to count 5-6-7-8!) No excuses. You just did it. You could sit there and watch and risk having her stern gaze lock eyes with you, or you could get out of the class. She had a serious no-bull-shit and no-bitches-in-my-class type of attitude. We all either loved her or hated her. She scared me.

I remember when she started choreographing partner pieces, in either groups of two or three. I remember freezing mid-routine. I remember feeling so defeated because I was so nervous I couldn't even remember two to eight seconds of motion. I even remember going home to a song called "Brother" where I cried my eyes out and felt like the most useless imposter trying to sit in that class and act like I belonged. All of "Ahmir's girls" had been with her for years. They all understood her cues. They all seemed to understand music. They had all developed half-decent skills and were able to "dance". Not wiggle your ass in a night club type of dance. I mean, if you were part of Ahmir's team, you could dance! I felt so painfully sub-standard. Always off count, delayed reactions, unable to stick to a count, unable to feel the music, unable to memorize steps. The amount of self-judgement that took place in my head was enough to erode the CN Tower. Yet, I observed how these older ladies kept coming back.

They couldn't possibly be in less pain than me after a class. There must have been far greater factors at play and it was only after two and a half years that I came to appreciate the heart that she put into every lesson. The camaraderie that was built was even deeper than any high school or varsity team because each person was there purely by their passion and accord. Each of us became famous for one reason or another. One lady was the ballet lady, she made every piece look soft and elegant. One was known as the super confident stewardess, she could make a rag look sexy. Another lady was known as "mama" because she had three sons. Another lady was known for being crazy because she had a wild and untamed sense of humor. As for myself, I was known as the forgetful one. I was always the first one to run out of RAM and couldn't remember steps. One of the most touching incidents was when we learned a three and a half minute routine and during the solo practice, I blanked out. My mind was just blank. As blank as a white board. I remember looking to the side of the room, my eyes in a desperate plea for help, when the entire squad hinted at a pirouette. I was so immensely touched I went home and cried that night. The loner in me didn't feel so alone anymore. I had friends. Ultra-supportive friends. They didn't care if I was forgetful, they only cared if I would continue. That was true friendship, people who accepted you for your flaws.

After two and a half years of training with this amazing instructor called Ahmir, she decided to part farewell with us. She had bigger plans and other ambitions outside of her teaching and dancing career. During one of her nearly last pieces of jazz choreography for the team, we had a number of insanely difficult combinations. Ahmir was at the point where it didn't matter what others thought, she had trained us like dancers and expected us to execute like dancers albeit a bit of a slow and forgetful dancer such as myself. The tune was "100% Pure Love". Vogueing and a double turn into splits in the middle of a routine! AAAARRRGGGGHHHH!!! Can you hear the squeak of dread in my voice? YES, a double pirouette straight into splits! Someone actually captured me doing that on camera. Otherwise I wouldn't even believe it was possible for me to do it. The sheer elation that I felt when I watched the video is hard to explain in words. There was just pure joy, a testimony that all the late nights of practicing with a full time job and as a single mom finally paid off! (Oh yes, I divorced somewhere along the journey....) Dancing provided me with a massive sense of growth and accomplishment. Something no other hobby has been able to do in all my years. The music, the emotions, the physical challenge, it's just the most enjoyable thing!

As with all art forms, there is no right or wrong. There is no perfection beyond the movement that took place in that very moment. Unless captured on video, a dancer's art and a dancer's gift is only there for a blink of an eye. For painters, sculptors, photographers, writers, work can be memorialized onto paper and passed on for generations. For dancers however, without the aids of modern technology and the oh-so-powerful iPhone camera, their work is a gift or immense dedication that is often highly undervalued.

Creativity is something each of us innately have within us, but very few people are often inspired enough to take action. Dancing for me has been a journey of self-rediscovery, a process of reconnecting with my soul and re-evaluating who I am and who I want to become. The energy that dancing moves through the body has been liberating, sometimes even orgasmic! Yeah, there, I said it - orgasmic. If you haven't had one in a while, it's time to go dance!

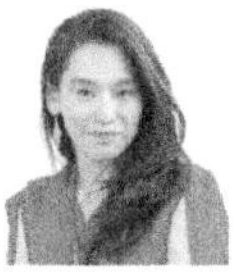

About Judy Wong

Judy Wong helps people all around the world become more confident, radiant, and effective by shifting their mindset to become more aligned with their true purpose.

As a public speaker and author Judy dedicates her time to empowering others to find greater fulfilment in their careers, create stronger deeper connections, and live more vibrantly while building greater prosperity. Her Amazon #1 Best Selling book on leadership, The Softer Side of the Corner Office was instrumental in helping other women recognize and avoid some of the common pitfalls of climbing the corporate ladder. As a corporate governance specialist, having worked on Wall Street and with executives for Fortune 500 companies across various industries and sectors on different continents, Judy has an eye for reputational and branding risks.

She has helped companies save millions of dollars by implementing the right strategies and protection mechanisms ahead of turbulent times. Along Judy's dedicated path towards personal development and expression, she was led towards artistic pursuits that opened her heart and mind to greater meaning and happiness. As a late-comer on to the stage, Judy's passion for dancing, writing and other forms of expression allows her to build strong connections with those who cross her path. Under the tutelage of world class mentors such as Bob Proctor, JT Foxx & Mark Anthony Bates, Judy openly shares her experiences and advice with audiences globally on her podcast Breaking The Glass Ceiling and through her life changing program, Magnetic Woman.

Judy is a firm believer in positively contributing to the grander evolution of humankind by helping others create a life that they are truly proud of. She specializes in strategies that are quick and easy for her clients to implement and master. Her results are proven and praised.

Connect with Judy at:

- Judywong.ascension@gmail.com
- www.facebook.com/judywywong
- www.instagram.com/judywywong
- http://ascension-development.mykajabi.com/

Past the Breaking Pointe

By Melissa Sullivan

"Let's move it! Girls, get on the stage now!" I heard the bellowing of my ballet instructor over the music coming from the piano on stage. We all scrambled to the wings, doing last minute limbering exercises to loosen up before we headed out onto the stage. I looked out past the curtain obscuring our positions and into the audience. There were just a handful of people out in the seats; after all, it was just a dress rehearsal. The stage lights shone brightly in my face as I looked up. After years of practice, bleeding toes, and sore muscles, I'd found my home at age thirteen. I could feel the music within my soul and dance into my own world, away from everyday distractions and worry, away from the bluntness of life. It was my safe zone; I could be me. The music stopped and startled me back to reality. This was my time, the moment. My instructor moved to the edge of the curtain, ready to count us out onto the stage. She gave us all a grin and I knew I was ready. The familiar and soothing sounds of Tchaikovsky began to rain upon the theatre. My heart skipped a beat as I made my entrance upon the stage.

All was well. I was home. They say home is where the heart is; it's a common phrase that feels like it's overused at times, but when it can apply to a situation, it provides comfort to those who utilize it. I actually have a pillow with those words strategically etched onto it. Home can be described as the place where you head back to after a long day of work, or the place that you consider to be your main place of residence, but it can mean something else also. It transcends time, space, and limitations. Home is where YOUR heart is. This is a place where you feel as though you have no limitation set on you. This is where you're at ease with what is going on and happy. It's all about being comfortable with who you are and where you are going.

For some people, home isn't a physical place. Home can be a feeling or even an action that makes a person feel like they are more like themselves. It took me some years to come to this conclusion. Although I had found an outlet early in life, I had also found negative emotions which fed into my insecurities and ran very deeply. My thoughts would spiral into places that I didn't think I'd go to, and my feelings would become something twisted and not of my own creation. "Escaping" seemed my only option for survival. I knew I needed an outlet which could provide something to relieve my mind of those negative thoughts and give me some sort of comfort in order to move forward with my life. When I danced on the stage, I felt as if I were escaping something; up until this point, I did not know what I was escaping from. I had always been an emotional child, full of imagination and wonder. I didn't understand why I felt different from other children. And early on, it didn't matter to me. I liked being different. Being imaginative allowed me to come up with amazing ideas that had me praised when I was younger and allowed my world to expand earlier than most children. But unfortunately, as life has a way of doing, it can sometimes wear down the youthful, independent soul within a child until it fades. Then, all that is left is how others expect people to act and behave. And it was during my college years that it began to take its toll.

I was a junior in college. I looked out my window and I saw a white woven blanket spread out before me. The snow that had started the day before draped itself upon the big oak trees outside my window. It was a beautiful scene. It was a thick, dry snow, the kind that crunches beneath your feet. I could feel the cold air through the window. Part of me wanted to stay inside and cozy up with a cup of hot cocoa while the other part wanted to head out into the snow and test just how crunchy it was.

I ended up turning back to my studies, but I couldn't help but feel homesick. I was stuck here; the snow had caused traffic issues and even though I had a car, I couldn't go anywhere that wasn't off campus. With that feeling of being trapped within me, I began to think about my time before college. I felt as if my dancing ability had declined because of my focus on my studies. I knew that my time at college took precedence, but there was a nagging feeling inside of me that wanted me to make sure that my dancing skills remained sharp. I felt hopeless and depressed; ballet had always given me the euphoria of feeling free as a bird. It took away my pains and regrets, if only for a little while. Only now, that feeling had all but disappeared. With the snow, it seemed as though my motivation for anything other than my studies was quashed. My escape plan had been crushed.

It was during that time that I knew I had to find another outlet. Since my college didn't offer a dance course, I had to find something else that would provide me with a creative outlet. Theatre filled the void. Majoring in theatre helped me to have the stage time I so loved. I was dancing a little during this time, but not to the degree I was accustomed to dancing. My theatre classes were based mostly on utilizing the stage as an actor, working the space as you went through your lines. It was a lot different from what I was used to and although I did enjoy aspects of it, it wasn't the same as being able to dance.

Being a theatre major was a very testing and emotional time period for me. Emotions are defined as a natural instinctive state of mind deriving from one's circumstances, mood, or relationships with others. There are too many emotions to name, but they can affect everyone in some way, shape, or form. I would say that during my childhood, I experienced a vast array of them, as most people do. When we are young, our emotions tend to dominate our thoughts if we feel strongly about something. It can take a while for a child to not be angry with someone if they feel they are slighted. Sadness can also affect children for days at a time, if the situation is personal. As was my case in particular, I grew up in a fear induced coma where I was constantly on edge or didn't quite "fit in." My fear encompassed a lot of the things I did that I wasn't comfortable with when I first tried them. I would have problems being introduced to new situations, as I'd be afraid that I'd mess something up or wouldn't be good at what I was asked to do.

After college, I decided to do what seemed normal in the eyes of my peers; get married and start a family. It was what was expected of me, and I didn't feel the need to fight against the norm. However, my marriage is something that I do not regret at all and it goes without saying that becoming a mother was the most powerful and wonderful thing that has ever happened to me. I was, for all intents and purposes, "settled." While getting used to my domestic life, I still felt the urge to dance again. My time was not my own, at that point. I had mouths to feed and children to take care of, so the time that I did have to myself wasn't focused on my own wants and needs. It did take some time for me to finally give myself the opportunity to dance again, not as a student, but as a teacher. Teaching students wasn't what I had planned for myself to continue my dancing, but it was an outlet that helped to fill that role. I was showing off the skills I had learned during my days as a dancer to a new generation of dancers. I worked with them to make sure that they were understanding the movements and knew that it wasn't going to be an easy process. When one of my students came to me, nearly in tears, that she had sores on her feet that were chafing against her pointe shoes, I had to explain that it was part of being a ballet dancer. It was going to hurt because her feet weren't used to the positions yet and she would be in pain, but if she truly enjoyed dancing, then the pain would fade with time.

Although I was teaching ballet, I certainly never saw myself as being an entrepreneur or owning my own studio. I had decided to go with the flow, and just live, letting my family and my teaching career dictate my life. And it worked, until it didn't. The anxious thoughts and depressed moods inched their way back into my life, even though I was using my dancing as a way of escape.

Motherhood was rewarding, but very intense, especially when there were three children running around begging for three different things! There was and still is, always something happening; the stress of my daily life then began to bleed into my teaching. I found that I was much more strict with my students because I was tense from my time at home. My husband did his best to make sure that I didn't feel alone in raising our children, but the stress of motherhood wasn't something easily pushed to the side. With three kids to worry about and care for, that part of my life began to take more precedence. My dance classes then began to seem like a chore; something that I had to go to teach instead of wanting to go to.

At this point in my life, however, I had not found a sufficient substitute to lessen the stress. I felt as if I was on a roller coaster, gripping the handle bars to keep from falling out as the hills and valleys rocked me in and out of my seat. Looking back, the image of me, holding my merlot in one hand, the vacuum cleaner in the other, all while watching the stove and the kids, seems absurd now. Still, it was my life at that time, and I had found it acceptable, normal, and the status quo. All the while, I kept telling myself, "I deserve some merlot after the day I've had," or, "everyone else enjoys a toddy for their motherly efforts." Taking the stress off with a drink seemed rational and made sense. I didn't get to the point where I was making excuses to drink, but if given more time, that would have been the road I'd have gone on.

What I hadn't expected, though, was that there was a better way. It took some time, but over the course of a few months, I began to make small changes. One, I would choose to meditate instead of reaching for the glass of merlot when things had become too overwhelming. I limited my drinks to only a few per week, then slowly whittled it down so that I wasn't drinking every day. Two, I would make sure I had enough time for a "me moment." This could be reading a chapter in a book or listening to music. I realized that even with teaching dance, I wasn't making the time for just myself; there was always someone else I needed to watch or take care of. Lastly, exercise became a key factor in my life. I had talked about doing ballet fitness with a few friends. I even taught a few classes outside of my normal ballet classes, but I wanted to be certified. The extra training and certification was very important to me. So, I began to look around.

I looked at other programs that offered quick certification for people who wanted to teach ballet, but none of them seemed thorough enough or the teachers didn't seem to care about what they were teaching. When I started to look for another alternative, the BalletBeFit Method immediately caught my eye. I liked how Rachel presented the program and felt she was hands on and would help in any way she could. She was personable and answered the questions I had about the class before I even registered. She made sure to explain everything so that I knew exactly what I was getting into. So, I signed up.

The journey so far has been amazing. If you would have told me a year and a half ago I would be working in a gym gaining clients and certified in Ballet Fitness, financially free and content, I would have not believed you! I owe it all to Rachel's teachings and the core aspects of BalletBeFit, as it helped me to get myself centered in a way that I hadn't been for a long time. Believe me, life is still hard and not always fair, but I've learned to live in the moment and not focus on what is behind nor in front of me. I focus on the now. My thoughts of going with the flow have been realized in a much more orderly way. The fears I had when beginning my classes have all but dissipated, since knowing that the future can change on a whim helps me to be more grounded in the "now" instead of the "later."

Life is about progress, not perfection and I try to instill this same life tool with my children as well. Teaching them to accept the things that happen in the moment without worrying about what will happen in the far future has hopefully helped them to not have the same crippling fear that I did when I was younger. Although the emotions are still there, I am able to identify them as feelings and feelings don't last. They come and go, both good feelings and bad feelings. If there are things that we need to hold onto, we will do so without holding onto the fleeting emotions that we had at the time.

What is important to remember is where your heart is rooted. What is it that you really want? How can you make a difference? These thoughts are good to meditate on, as they can provide insight into how you wish to live your life. These questions don't have simple answers, so taking the time to unpack them will benefit you greatly in the future. As long as I'm grounded in myself and do the right thing next, I am able to answer those questions with confidence and perseverance. I may not have the complete answer to them, but I know that I will find it. Just remember that as we build up and empower one another, we are all just perfectly imperfect.

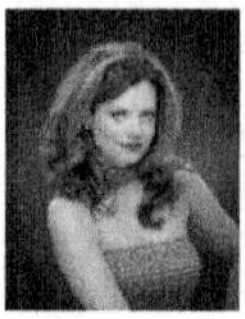

About Melissa Sullivan

Melissa Dunn Sullivan began her dance training at the age of six. She studied summers on scholarship with Ballet Austin under the direction of Stephen Mills, Ballet Mississippi under Jullian Davis, and the Atlanta Ballet. She has taken master classes with David Howard, Tom Clower, and Anne Burton Avery.

Once graduating high school, Melissa attended Belhaven College on scholarship where she was a member of Ballet Magnificat's pre-professional training division under the direction of George Lysenko. She was offered an apprenticeship position to dance professionally with Ballet Arkansas under the direction of Kurt Hathaway.

Melissa has over twenty years of experience teaching ballet, tap, and lyrical dance (ages 3-adult.) She has danced numerous roles, including Lilac Fairy with Ballet Dallas, Sugar Plum Fairy, Arabian princess, Dewdrop, and Snow Queen in the Nutcracker. Other full length ballets include Coppelia and Cinderella.

She was Ballet Mistress and board member for the Tupelo Ballet as well as a member of the MS Dance Association and is currently a board member for The Civic Ballet. She is a dance instructor for NMDC. She is working on her

Master's degree in English and resides in Saltillo with her three children.

Connect with Melissa at:

- yempowered12@gmail.com
- https://www.facebook.com/melissa.d.sullivan.7
- https://instagram.com/masullivan1?r=nametag
- https://www.classically-fit.com/

Looking Within

By Cadence Dollive

For this story I will start not at the beginning but in the middle...

It is 2009 and I am a newly qualified teacher (NQT) about to start my first job at a fabulous all girls' school. The moment I had walked through the front gates of this school for my interview I knew I wanted to work here, everything about it just felt right, and to have got the job was the most amazing boost to my confidence. I felt excited and nervous all at the same time as I walked into the classroom to meet the group of students who would be my Form group for the year. I was met with smiling faces all willing to offer me help and answer any of my questions, they put me at ease and in that moment I felt I had made the right decision for my career.

Fast forward a few years to 2013, for weeks now I have arrived home and immediately set to getting ready for another school day, I eat while I work, and hours later my eyes grow tired as I stare unproductively at a set of students' work I am trying to mark ready for a lesson tomorrow, the words seem to swim away out of focus and I can barely read what they have written. My mind drifts distracted to other tasks on my ever growing 'to do' list and the extra responsibilities I have taken on in school also weigh on my mind. I have just a few more books to mark but it is getting so late I must concede defeat. I lie awake for ages, feeling frustrated as my head spins with too many thoughts as I try to get to sleep. This has been getting worse for more than twelve months and now I am thinking perhaps teaching is not the right career for me. Back to the true beginning:

The child mind.

Working with young people is a privilege, their optimism and enthusiasm is infectious, and it always amazes me how they manage to achieve so many fabulous things whether it be speaking several languages or playing several instruments, performing on stage, representing sporting teams or raising money for charity to name but a few. Nothing seems to stand in their way, if they believe they can do it, more often than not they will. When I look back at my own childhood I can see how my mind worked in a different way to how I think now, I didn't see barriers, only opportunities. As a child I was very focused and some might say stubborn, in my world if I wanted to achieve something I would just get on and do it with my Taurean determination and perseverance. While at school I took part in and achieved lots of things, I really loved school. I did pretty well academically, played sports, played the flute, attended orchestra, performed in concerts, and then there was my passion for horses.

In a recent conversation with my mum I asked her when she thought I first developed a love of horses, and she told me of a photograph she had found of me when I was two years old. We had been on holiday to the Isle of White and while we were there, I had my first ride on a donkey. My mum told me that, unlike some of the other young children, I had shown no fear and as soon as I had sat on the donkey my face had lit up with joy. For my fifth birthday I started to have regular riding lessons once every two weeks. I loved riding more than anything, and even if the weather was too bad to ride, I would enjoy just being at the stables, around the horses grooming their soft coats and feeling the warmth of their breath on my face. Being around horses for me was the most magical experience and I soon became obsessed.

I would constantly daydream about them, I would read books about girls who found and rescued ponies and trained them up to then compete at local shows winning clear round competitions, my imagination would run wild as I pictured myself doing the same. Whilst many adults in my life speculated this love of horses would come to an end once I reached my teens, I started planning for my future being a horse owner. As soon as I could start earning pocket money I was saving all I could. I also made sure I could be around horses as much as possible and started working weekends at my local riding school for which I was rewarded with free rides. After years of mucking out, and saving any money I bought my first horse by age fifteen. He was the most wonderful companion to me and owning him for the three and a half years also taught me lots of valuable lessons. Having come from a non-horsey family and background he was my full responsibility, so I had to step up to the job. I quickly learned lots about time management as I had to fit in looking after and riding him around my school work and orchestra rehearsals, I also learned to budget as I only had what money I had left from what I had saved to buy him. In those few years we formed the most amazing bond and as the time came nearer for me to sell him as I got ready to go to University I was heartbroken. His final lesson for me was about letting go, so I could move onto the next stage in my life as I began working out my career path. At the stage I had no clear idea what I wanted to do with my life, but there was at least one thing I was certain of, I knew I needed to have horses in my life, always.

What do you want to be?

'What do you want to be when you grow up?' A fun question to ask children. I'm certain I changed mine by the minute "farmer, astronaut, vet, explorer, detective, mermaid!" At a young age this question is a fun way of finding out more about a child's interests and I quite enjoyed thinking of what I might be. As I moved on through my education this seemingly innocent question started to have a more serious and permanent emphasis as school and college began to demand of me an answer. I am going to be a....?

As I came to choose my 'A' levels the number of people asking me this question seemed to increase and I would be given lists which appeared to contain more jobs than there are stars in the sky which was less than helpful. I quickly began to envy those who are born with the innate knowledge that they are going to be a lawyer or a doctor or whatever career they have fixed their compass point to. I had, of course looked into what I loved doing which took me to options enabling me to work with horses, however, after spending some valuable time at various equestrian facilities for work experience I couldn't see a career for myself working at a yard as a groom, or at a riding school which at the time seemed to be the only options being suggested to me. I now began to look to my other interests such as music and animals. I already had achieved my grade 8 in flute, but I didn't feel drawn to a career as a musician, so I narrowed my ideas down to something involving animals but again the only options that kept coming my way were vet or vet nurse, these seemed like not a bad idea so I choose sensible 'A' levels which would potentially enable me to enter this area of work. Whilst studying for my 'A' levels, further work experience highlighted that being a vet was also not for me. My other interest was the natural world,

I have always enjoyed being in nature. I had been lucky enough to grow up in the Yorkshire countryside and enjoyed taking long walks with my grandad pretty much as soon as I could walk. My grandparents loved wildlife, especially birds and this love of nature soon rubbed off on me. A friend of mine had gone to University to study Zoology and the more I found out about the course I decided it was for me, so I was thrilled to gain a place to study Zoology at the University of Manchester. Not an obvious choice of subject to lead into a specific career, and most people I spoke to assumed this would lead me to working in a zoo, which to be honest I am sure I would enjoy too. I really enjoyed studying for my degree despite some health issues along the way, but on completing my course I still had no specific direction I wanted to take my life in.
Then along came an opportunity which would change

everything. Whilst I was completing my final university exams a friend of mine had gone to work at a summer camp in America and suggested it would be something I would enjoy, so I looked it up online and really liked the look of it as I would be able to get back to riding, which I had missed while at University, so I went ahead and applied. During this time I also started planning to travel with another friend and soon the date to fly to America arrived.

Teaching at the summer camp was without a doubt one of the best experiences of my life. I met so many amazing people and the experience also increased my confidence and self-esteem. I have always struggled with self-belief so to have made it to America on my own was a big achievement. My main role at camp was caring for the camp's horses in the morning and then teaching riding lessons to campers throughout the day, along with loads of other activities to get involved in. There were so many opportunities to try new things, and I made some amazing friends along the way, some of whom I would see again very soon on my travels through Australia and New Zealand. I will be forever grateful for this experience which taught me the value of stepping out of my comfort zone and the benefit of taking risks. Having never done anything like this on my own before I was incredibly nervous but then felt proud of myself for negotiating these challenges. It was also whilst at camp that I started to feel that a job in education might be a possible career, I really enjoyed teaching and working with the campers. I started to feel that maybe being a teacher might be a possible career, the experience also reminded me how much being around horses made me happy, they have such a calming influence on me, being around them is genuinely a kind of therapy for me.

Not long after camp had finished I flew back to the UK and within a few days my bags were repacked. I met my friend at the airport and we set off to visit Cambodia, Singapore, Malaysia, Australia and New Zealand. It was another incredible adventure which again gave my confidence a much-needed boost. Looking back now I am so grateful to the people who made these opportunities possible for me. Having decided whilst traveling that I was going to train to be a teacher, not long after my return to the UKin 2008 I began my teacher training course.

Where do you see yourself in.....?

I was never under any illusion that a career in teaching was going to be easy, my mum had worked in a high school as an art technician so many of her friends were teachers whom she had seen struggle with the stresses of the job. However, I still felt I wanted to give it a go. I managed very well through my teacher training and landed my first job as an NQT at a private Girls' School. I quickly learned if there is one job which certainly needs 'adaptable, energetic, enthusiastic' in the job description it is teaching. For example you might plan a lesson which goes amazing with one class and think you have nailed it then teach the same lesson with another class and it just doesn't work out at all, you leave the classroom scratching your head wondering how this could be. I enjoy the challenge of making my lessons engaging and accessible, so I decided I wanted to further my own education and embarked on a Masters in Education at the University of Huddersfield whilst still working full time. Although I was usually really good at time management, I was beginning to struggle, as I was still new to my teaching role. I sometimes struggled to prioritise things correctly, especially when something like an email would arrive in my inbox out of the blue which appeared to need dealing with immediately, yet I didn't feel I had the time. I was finding all of this very challenging and I started to struggle with anxiety as the different demands on my time and energy began to wear me down.

To add to the stress, having decided on my career path there was now a new question to consider 'where do you see yourself in 1, 3, 5, 10 years?'... erm? Panic! I once again felt the pressure to find an answer and again I began to envy the individuals who had their lives mapped out in front of them. I am sure some people who join the teaching profession see themselves working up the career ladder and eventually becoming a Head of Department or Head teacher, but not me, I just wanted to be a great teacher but I began to feel like this wasn't the right attitude and I must want to 'progress'. Being driven by these external cue's I began to put myself under pressure to follow the well trodden paths of careers in teaching. In order to try and fit in with these expectations I took on a role of responsibility in school. It very quickly became apparent to me that this was not the right job for me, but I could only think of how bad it would look if I didn't at least try and make it work, so I decided to stick with it and give it a go. I had lots of excellent support and worked closely with a colleague I consider my friend, however, this role felt entirely the wrong fit for me. This was to be the beginning of things starting to unravel for me as details of who I was and what I wanted to be, began to fray and I held onto trying to make a success of this role. I put pressure on myself to 'not fail' but as I became more overwhelmed and exhausted I also became less productive. I felt tired all of the time and had no energy to give to others, leading to the daily confusion and tangled mess of incomplete work, stress and anxiety. I began to lose confidence in my ability to do my job and developed a negative mindset around work.

My creativity suffered as I was unable to focus on anything and eventually I began to have bouts of anxiety and panic attacks which I hid from people as I felt ashamed. Talking about mental health issues was and, although things are improving, still is stigmatised. I felt guilty for asking for people's time or help as I felt they had their own and more pressing problems to deal with and I didn't want to bother them with mine. Also, to be honest, I didn't really understand what was going wrong. As I continued to struggle on, I began thinking that maybe teaching wasn't the right career for me. But I had at one point loved teaching, and I was determined to see if I could find this love for my job again. The one thing that held my last few threads together was my horse, who I had bought after my first year as a teacher, so at the end of each stressful and exhausting day, he was my constant support and stability and also my therapy, with him I could just be me.

Prioritise yourself to serve others

*"It's what you do in the dark that puts you in the light" - **Michael Phelps***

I was broken, and when you break something is forced to change. I did eventually get to the stage where I felt so lost and overwhelmed I admitted defeat and handed in my notice on the extra role of responsibility hoping this would be the end of my problems. The initial relief was overwhelming so I knew I had made the right decision, however it wasn't the whole solution I hoped it would be, ultimately I had lost my confidence and my self esteem was at an all time low, and most damaging of all I had lost my direction and purpose.

This was the start of a huge learning curve as I now began looking inwards in order to reset my course to navigate towards finding myself again. One of the first things which enabled me to do this was picking up a book my mum had bought me called 'Quiet' by Susan Cain. It had been sitting on my bookshelf for a year or two and finally over a summer break I started to read. Straight away I began to recognise some of the reasons for the fatigue and exhaustion I was experiencing. I learned that as I am an introvert, as much as I enjoy being around people this drains my energy. This explained why I was so exhausted by the end of the day with so many, sometimes more than a hundred, people requiring my energy and attention and support each day. I learned why jobs and projects which really interest and resonate with me would be easy for me to focus on, and even give me energy and motivate me, whereas others which were less aligned with my interests and beliefs would drain my energy and have a negative effect on my health. This explained why I struggled so much with taking on the extra role in school. I had known at the start it wasn't right and I should have listened to my intuition.

On finishing 'Quiet' I wanted to learn more, I still had a long way to go and needed to start learning to trust my intuition and rebuild my confidence, but where to start? Once I started looking it didn't take long to find more reading material, TED talks and podcasts all relating to finding your purpose, dealing with anxiety and rebuilding confidence. The next lesson I learned the importance of prioritising myself to ensure I had enough energy to give others the attention they needed and deserved. It was now that I started to put some of this advice into practice. I started small by making seemingly inconsequential alterations to my daily routine. One of the first things I did for myself was I started making sure I took my vitamins every morning, a simple act of self-care I had previously neglected. Also I made sleep a priority as this was one area where I knew if I was tired I would quickly become irrational, irritable, less productive and more likely to have anxiety or a panic attack. I also scheduled at least fifteen minutes each night to read as this calmed my mind and ensured I had better quality sleep It amazed me how quickly I began to see the benefits from making small, sustainable changes to my routine. As the weeks went on these changes became second nature and I began to feel my energy returning and my mood began to improve. Over the coming months I continued to try different things such as scheduling in time each week, sometimes just ten minutes on an evening for activities such as yoga, reading or walking.

Making work, work for you

"All you have to decide is what to do with the time that is given to you" - ***Gandalf***

My routine at home was working to help me manage my anxiety and feel more prepared for each day, however my anxiety could still be triggered by unpredictable and last minute requests happening during the day. I had started the helpful habit of planning no more than four key tasks I had to complete each day, but on most days these plans could quickly fall apart when I suddenly needed to fit an important phone call, reply to an email, meet with a student, into an already packed teaching day. The reason this increased my anxiety was the feeling that I had to act immediately to the request which I understand is a pressure I put on myself. This would send me into a bit of a spin, as I was now trying to fit into my day more than was feasible, this would leave me with the feeling that I hadn't given anyone or anything my full attention or dealt with the situation to the best of my ability. On top of all of that I would finish the day still having work I had planned to get done in the day left to do in the evening leaving little time for myself and once again I started to feel tired and frustrated. Just as things were starting to get on top of me again it was a conversation with the author of this book in which I was expressing my frustration that she happened to give me one of the most helpful pieces of advice I have ever been given. She suggested that first I ensure I schedule in a period of time each day (even just ten minutes) which is assigned to dealing with any such events which may require my immediate attention. She also advised that I should set some clearer boundaries, so rather than trying to react to a request for a phone call or reply to an email in full straight away, reply to them with a view to scheduling in time later in the week for a phone call or explain you will get back to them by a specific time, not only does this take away the immediate pressure to respond, but also gives your thinking time and means you give your full attention to the task or person you are talking to. I started applying this advice and I quickly began to see the benefits to this way of working.

I was able to schedule calls and meetings around my work commitments for each day so I was completing everything to a much better standard. I started being able to leave work each day having accomplished all or at least the majority of what I had set out to do, this has made the biggest difference to my overall routine, productivity and job satisfaction and more time to focus on the things that are important to me and my health and wellbeing.

Look back to see forward

The biggest benefit of all of these small changes combined is I was able to find myself and my purpose once again. During my more challenging times I would describe them as dark, lonely and a feeling of being lost. It is quite scary feeling like this as you don't know in what direction to turn. The small changes I made, especially those which prioritised my self care enabled my childhood passions for learning, music, wildlife and reading to find their way back into my life. With my renewed energy I started to create activities which played to my strengths and my interests such as running the school equestrian team, science reading challenges for students and projects to help local wildlife. My enthusiasm also returned to my teaching having spent time prioritising myself and my interests I had gained better insight into who I am and what I can offer and what projects and roles would benefit myself and others.

The main lesson I have learned is that we all have something unique to offer and when you find it, it will bring you joy and fulfilment and hopefully benefit others somehow too. Having someone come to you and thank you for something only you could have done is one of the most rewarding feelings, as you know you have made a positive difference to that person. When students come to me now to tell me how well they did on their horse in a school team event, or to discuss a book they have read on one of the science reading challenges I have put together brings me joy. I have learned how by following your own path and turning up as you, is the way to have the most positive outcomes not only for yourself but for others also. I am incredibly lucky to work at a school which encourages this and has enabled me to keep following and developing my interests and passions. I now enjoy that I am still a work in progress, but as I look back I can now connect the dots to where I am now and begin to see more clearly where I want to be in the future by looking to what I love and am passionate about making me more confident in navigating my own life path. Throughout my teaching journey so far there has been one individual who even in the darkest of times has brought some light back into my day and that is my horse. Horses for me are incredibly special animals, they are intelligent and no matter how bad my day has been spending time with them gives me time back to think and reflect and find myself once again, or if needed an ear to listen and a soft coat to cry into. As well as negotiating my teaching career, I have achieved my aim of having my own horse to compete and we have enjoyed success in showjumping and dressage competitions and still have lots of new and wonderful experiences to look forward to together.

Final thoughts:

If you find yourself in the dark remember there is always a way out, make small sustainable changes and your light will begin to shine through.

Be a work in progress and never stop learning, if you think you have all of the answers, pick up another book, listen to another podcast.

Be authentic, only you can offer something unique.

Prioritise yourself, you cannot be productive or of service to others if you are exhausted. Set boundaries and you your friends, family, colleagues and all in your life will benefit.

Hold on to your passions, they are what gives us our purpose and strength to keep fighting.

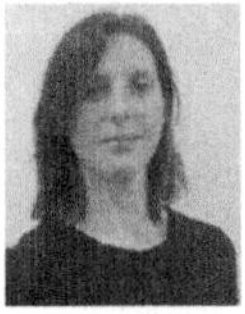

About Cadence Dollive

Cadence Dollive is a Biology teacher at a high school for girls', and has an MA in education. She is a strong believer in everyone having the freedom and opportunities to find and follow their own path and purpose in life, and delights in guiding and helping students on their own journeys. As a Zoology graduate from the University of Manchester, Cadence takes a keen interest and active role in promoting awareness of environmental issues and believes we all have a part to play in protecting the planet.

Cadence is a keen reader and promotes the benefits of reading to students through her programme of Science Reading Challenges. The aim being to broaden students' horizons and foster ideas and philosophies which they may not otherwise meet in their routine education.

As an Equestrian, Cadence has had success competing in both showjumping and dressage in the UK and believes in the benefits of being around animals for improving our physical and mental health and wellbeing. She uses her personal experiences and expertise to encourage and help others wishing to get the most from their partnership with horses.

Connect with Cadence at:

- cadence.dollive@balletbefit.com

Step Across Your Start Line

By Stephanie Bouvard

The truth is we will all cross our finish line at some stage but only a few of us consciously choose to cross our very own start line. This is a journey about how you can create your very own unique start line, swap chasing dreams for living dreams.

Do you ever catch yourself day dreaming or wondering what if? What if you had turned left instead of right? What if you had said no instead of yes? I know I did, and in fact I still do on the rare occasion. If I were to ask you what the link is between New York, Ballet, Running and Wine, you might think these are just some activities or holiday concepts, but to me these are the pillars of my daily life which were once just a fantasy but have become my reality. Yes, when I was growing up, I used to dream of ballet dancing in New York, when I was a young adult I used to dream of moving to New York and living by Central Park, as a runner I used to fantasize over the New York Marathon, and as I got older and started to appreciate wine I started dreaming about becoming a Master of Wine. Well, what if i told you that as I am typing this I am sitting in my New York apartment, three blocks away from Central Park, staring at my five New York City Marathon finisher medals, sipping a cup of coffee in between teaching a BalletBeFit class, coaching a group of runners for their next marathon and preparing my next blind wine tasting exam, would you believe me?

Yes, dreams do become your reality, if and only if you choose to draw your very own roadmap and cross your start line. I want to share with you my secret sauce and sizzle to making this happen for you but let's first rewind a little and place everything back into context. Follow me and you will see...

The time is 2013 and I'm standing in the start corrals of the World Major Tokyo Marathon. I've never run a marathon before, in fact only until about a year ago I hadn't really run more than about 10km continuously; quite frankly for a broad portion of my life running had always felt like a bit of a drag. I knew it was good for fitness and all that jazz, but I used to find it really tough to just have to run, breathe and deal with my thoughts (funnily enough as I tell you this am thinking "wow, bliss, all you have to do is left foot, right foot, breathe and have time to think? Sounds aw-maze-ing!!" right?!) So how did I get here? I had a right epiphany moment in 2010 and was swept off my feet, quite literally: as I was sweeping around my living room on a Saturday afternoon doing that weekly clean while singing and dancing my heart out, I jumped up to do a pirouette only to land with a bang and crash to the ground. I crashed so hard it crumbled my bones. Fast forward hours spent in the emergency room, x-rays and MRIs the verdict hit: I had a triple stress triple fracture in my left foot, had also torn and ripped tendons and ligaments in my ankle. Physically broken I was. Everything started to become blurry, the doctor was explaining that he could perform reconstructive surgery and started showing me different methods and prices, trying to convince me that this was all necessary if I didn't want to spend the rest of my life hobbling around with a permanent limp. Sadly I lived in Singapore, worked for a start up and had the worse health insurance in the world so there was not a chance I would be able to afford the reconstructive surgery required to heal this injury, my credit cards were maxed out from all the imagery costs. I had no choice but to accept this hard new reality. I just felt completely numb, hopeless and helpless, like I had suddenly lost myself. The doctor looked at me "well let's just say it's a good thing you're not a runner and you don't run marathons because you're definitely never running one of those in your life, in fact don't even think about running across the street to catch a bus, the impact will be too much and you will end up back in here without the choice but to have that surgery" . I was bubbling with anger frustration and deceit. My face was so hot, my heart started beating and pounding. Well maybe I wasn't a professional runner, and maybe I had never run a marathon, and maybe I had, had mixed feelings about running in the past but I suddenly felt the urge to run!

One thing I knew hadn't changed was that no one was ever going to tell me what I could or could not do, no one would have the right to ever decide whether or not I would be able to do something if I set myself out to achieve that. Determined I became, with a strong desire to not be defined by my failure and to prove I could do what others thought I was incapable of. A lot of my so called friends had always said I would never have the patience for long distance running, I wouldn't have the discipline to train for so long, they used to say I was too much of a fast and furious quick wins short term junky. Was this suddenly the test of life? The right of passage I needed to prove my worth? Why was this happening?

I hobbled out of the medical practice holding onto my crutches, backpack making my way to my apartment... only to discover my partner had walked out with all of my belongings. Emotionally broken I became. I wanted to bury myself into my work to forget about it all, but I was worn out, exhausted and felt like a gigantic open wound vulnerable to the world. I needed to take some time off to heal, I reached out to my boss and explained that I would not go on a business trip that week and would work remotely.

"No problem" he said. Finally, someone who supports me. I felt a little wave of relief until my phone beeped: it was my boss asking me to pop into the office for a "quick and easy meeting" , " the sooner the better" it said... somehow I made up this beautiful positive scenario where my colleagues would be taking the workload from me and my boss would be giving me paid leave to recover... When I got to the office no one was there to greet me, I had to crawl my way up one of those very steep shop house staircases, as I had barely caught my breath at the top I was waiting for me holding a letter. "Steph, thanks for coming in, I have made it really easy for you, I typed your resignation letter up and all you need to do is sign here"

I read the letter which basically was saying that I needed to quit because I was no longer fit to do my job. I was horrified and refused to sign. In return I received threats. That moment destroyed me even further. As an expat I knew I had ten business days to find a new job justifying my presence in Singapore or else I would get deported... that and all the bills and rent I had to pay...I signed, sobbed, and hobbled back to my apartment.

There I was standing amidst a world full of emptiness with nothing left to hold onto. Not fit for the job, not fit to run, not fit for Love... the irony hit me: how can I be so unFIT for everything when I have also been a fitness instructor for the past thirteen years? Something was not adding up here, for the very first time in my life, I actually needed a moment to sit still with my thoughts. Yes, for once I actually wanted to be in the present focusing on my breathing and letting myself go deep within. Looking and being fit had always been part of my journey, my identity, fit simply defined who I was. Suddenly being told that I was no longer fit and being put in front of the fact that I was not fit to do, to give, to receive, to accomplish, to achieve, to execute, was probably the hardest realization I was ever forced to make in life. That's when it hit me: my focus had always been on "looking fit" but not really "being fit". I was fit on the outside but in truth I really wasn't fit at all on the inside. Having suffered from bulimia nervosa since the age of eight, I had a very toxic relationship with food and my body image. Binging, purging, starving myself and over exercising were part of my daily routine and regime. I never nurtured my body, instead I would have negative thoughts about myself constantly "too fat, too bloated, too much this not enough that" ... the negative self talk voice was a constant. Constantly using exercise as a punishment for over eating and over eating using exercise as a license to eat. As I looked deeper within I tried to take stock of what was there: raw rashes and open wounds; was my eczema a way my body had had to externalize these rashes? It was time to heal, time to really dig deep into my soul, understand triggering events, understand what my soul really wanted me to see but overall understand who my heart and soul truly wanted me to be. This was the moment of epiphany: learn who I was.

Going through this soul searching process I noticed while I was internally intoxicated with anger and negative self talk, externally I always fought the battle of optimism and positivity: a firm believer the sun will shine tomorrow, after the rain comes the sun. Wow, it clicked: this positive outlook was always about waiting and hoping for things to pass or get better, but never about learning to dance in the storm or making lemonade with lemons.

If there was ever a perfect time to change, this was it. I started working with a psychiatrist and physical therapist, I thought that's what I "had" to do, a doctor for the body and a doctor for the soul. Soon enough I was back on my feet at the gym, I was jogging a little, got a new job, new friends, new apartment and met the love of my life. On the outside I "had it all", ticking all the boxes of a successful senior executive living in a huge condo with pool, gym, housekeeper, weekend champagne brunches, designer clothes, weekly beach week ends away...

Yet something was still missing. The relationship to my body and to food were still a constant daily battle, while I was able to identify triggers and have a couple of coping mechanisms, I could tap into I still wasn't there. I still wasn't madly in love with myself and I really still was suffering from eczema, allergies and bulimia. Let's face it I hadn't healed. I had simply thrown a band aid on my internal wounds, I was loading up on antihistamines, cortisone and Xanax but I hadn't truly deeply and most profoundly healed myself. I'd gone for that quick fix. And that doctor's voice in my head still frequently echoing "you will never run a marathon". I was thinking about this while browsing online planning my next trip to Tokyo I "accidentally" clicked on a banner which took me to the Tokyo marathon registration page and just like that I signed up. I felt a sudden rush of adrenaline, I felt in control in a weird way I had never felt in my life, was I feeling empowered or possessed I don't know but it was a feeling I was ready to embrace, channel and let me propel me into my future.

My husband came home and I said "I am going to run the Tokyo marathon!" "that's amazing I am so proud of you" he replied. Wow! he wasn't even doubting whether I could do it, he was already in the win. My brain suddenly went into type A planning mode: training, packing, logistics etc. the fitness instructor in me was suddenly struck by physiology principles: fueling, hydration, nutrition. What would I tell a client who was refusing to digest food yet wanted to run twenty six point two miles? I knew I was putting myself in danger. That was the moment when I took a hundred day pledge with myself that by day one hundred I would have made complete peace with my body, with food and would have crossed the Tokyo Marathon finish line.

It was time to get to work on my mindset and detoxifying my soul and my gut. Let me tell you it was not an easy process. I would spend hours staring at a bowl of pasta trying to eat it all up because I knew I had to go on a fifteen mile training run the next morning. Time to bring the big guns out: I ditched the psychiatrist, changed physical therapists, hired a naturopath and a yoga teacher. I needed a holistic approach if I really wanted to heal and change, this was going to be a full body-mind-nutrition-hydration-sleep journey. My yoga teacher taught me about yin restorative yoga, she taught me to reconnect with my heart, helped me see my inner strength and she helped me make peace with my body and my mind. My naturopath helped me understand what my body was truly craving for, she helped me work through my allergies, assisting me in healthy detox.

In turn I was able to gain a deeper knowledge of myself, identifying foods that served me and those that didn't. I discovered new forms of nutrition, found that carbs were not the enemy and plants could be a great source of protein. I realized that sleeping four hours a day didn't work for me and I was actually a nine hour sleeper. I learned how to read relationships and let go of those that consumed me.

Through this process I was able to reconnect with my dreams and my passion. My passion for movement, happiness and well being. My love for taking others on a journey with me. My dreams of living in New York and teaching Ballet. My fantasy of running the New York Marathon.

I had become committed to putting myself first. I quit my super career in marketing and advertising and went back to school. I took certifications in nutrition, wellness for women, running, exercise rehabilitation therapy, BalletBeFit, Yoga and Pilates. I was rebuilding myself and setting the foundations to make my dreams a reality. No this was not easy, it took a lot of work, dedication, commitment and discipline. I trained for the Tokyo Marathon alone, applying what I was learning through my education. Saying it was tough is an understatement, but everything was centered on being at ease and at peace with myself. All I knew is I wanted to get to that finish line not only alive, in one peace but most importantly feeling strong and confident, that was the focus.

The race itself was gruelling and I was probably the only runner downward-dogging it at mile eighteen!! I cried, I laughed, I sang, I screamed, I power talked to myself during the entire distance. When I took that right turn and saw the finish line the rush of adrenaline came back and I knew this was it: as I crossed the 2013 World Major Tokyo Marathon I realized that in this very moment I had just crossed my very own Start Line:

- I had let go of the shadow of the old,
- I had built self confidence and self belief,
- I was madly in love with my body for what it had just accomplished,
- I was finally healed and ready for my life to begin.

Tears of joy, pride, exhaustion and exhilaration were pouring out of my body, of my heart, of my soul. I still get shivers of excitement even as I speak about this today. I am so proud of what I was able to achieve through this journey because it literally revolutionized my life:

- I had finally developed an understanding of myself,
- I had left a career I had lost passion for and traded it in to helping others go through similar cathartic journeys.

The complete turning point was when my husband and I decided it was time to leave Singapore as I took an immense leap of faith in myself: I decided to start my own online and in person fitness & wellness business in New York where I have now been coaching runners for the New York City Marathon since 2017 but most importantly beyond crossing the NYCM finish line I have been helping hundreds of men and women cross their very own unique start line and this has been a gift! Back into my Manhattan living room I now want to share with you my secret sauce and sizzle to ignite your power, this helped me, and since has helped hundreds of others so I am confident there is something for you too: Five steps so you can cross your very own start line:

1. Describe your dream in detail and explain it: I find the more you explain and talk about your dream the more real it becomes.

2. Make peace with yourself, your body, your mind, food, people; you need your energy to be constructive not destructive.

3. Take a pledge and hold yourself accountable: honestly without that pledge I took with myself on January 1st 2013 I never would be where I am today.

4. Find your mentors, your supporters and your fans: be inspired and inspire others but also learn when to let go of relationships that will only consume you.

5. Committed, disciplined with a sprinkle of flexibility: we've all heard the saying "Rome wasn't built overnight" well executing a dream is no one night stand either, everything you do and think should be pointing towards that same direction you are aiming at while at the same time remaining open minded and open hearted for opportunities that may arise along the way.

If you apply these five steps as a result you will ignite your super power so you can step out of your shell to step into your shine and inspire the world to cross their start line too!!

Now you may ask what's next for me? Well I am still loving what I do everyday, because as we all know when you do what you love and you love what you do you don't work a single day but rather fulfil your life everyday. For me that's coaching runners, teaching BalletBeFit classes and working on a passion project around wine, vines and oenology, but that's definitely a story for another day...

Laugh and Sweat Everyday, be at ease and at peace.

With Love,
Coach StephB

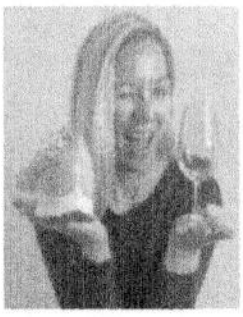

About Stephanie Bouvard

Stephanie Bouvard-Moreton also known as Coach StephB is a Franco-British New York based fitness professional and plant powered wine expert. Steph coaches female runners in their forties and beyond. She is notorious for her knowledge in physiology and anatomy which grant her an eagle eye for runners' biomechanics. In addition, her areas of expertise are deeply rooted in a holistic approach to wellness and fitness: mobility, strength, nutrition and mindset.

Coach Steph started her fitness career as a group exercise instructor back in the late nineties as a part time job while at university. Upon graduating with distinction from a Master's degree in International Business from the Grenoble Graduate School of Business, France, she then moved into a career of sports marketing and media while still keeping a part time gig in personal training. It wasn't until 2013 that she decided it was time to live fully her passion: help women love their body through the powers of running. She quit her corporate job as a global marketing VP and went full throttle into coaching. It was then that she studied closer the human body and worked alongside physical therapists and naturopaths so she could better support her clients to run and live pain free both physically and mentally.

Most recently Steph reconnected with ballet and became the first US based fit-pro to be certified to teach

BalletBeFit, a unique form of exercise which uses ballet principles and fitness modalities. Steph teaches a ballet inspired strength and mobility class specifically designed for women who like to run.

Stephanie is also extremely passionate about wine and at time of writing was preparing to take on the grueling Advanced Diploma in Wine with the Wine & Spirit Education Trust. Steph strongly believes that Wellness doesn't mean Wineless and thus wants to support women who have a strong desire to invest in their wine and their well-being.

When not designing a class, coaching a group of runners or revising for a blind wine tasting exam, you will find Steph cooking up a feast in the kitchen while discussing the next family adventure with her husband Paul and their two fur-babies (the Furbies) Yuki and Nushka. The four of them are inseparable and go absolutely everywhere together!

To connect with Steph go to her personal website www.coachstephb.com where you can access her coaching services, fit-pro mentoring opportunities and private wine investment solutions. She is very responsive and will be happy to hear from you!

Connect with StephB at:

- https://www.sommstephb.com/
- wine@sommstephb.com
- training@coachstephb.com
- www.coachstephb.com

Don't Wait To Glow Your Best

By Rebecca Landy

I have heard the excuses that keep people from doing what they want said time and time again from clients, family members, and even myself. There's always tomorrow, next week, when the kids get older, when there's more money in my account, when I have more time...the list goes on and on. We limit ourselves to what we're able to do at a single point in time and may put off the things that can allow us to lead a richer life. The key is to remove those excuses and take chances on the experiences that will help you to lead a fulfilling life.

My goal is to help you glow your best, allowing your inner self that has no doubts or concerns to emerge and achieve what you might not have thought possible.

I won't lie; it's taken me most of my life to develop this process. This is not a one-size-fits-all approach either, so many of the skills I want to share with you might not resonate as much as others will. That's okay; my goal is, at the very least, to have you thinking about your own way to get yourself glowing. I don't know where you are on your journey of self-discovery. Even if you haven't even thought about the process, it can be a bit overwhelming to just get into the thick of it and start to glow right away. For some people, they need to have a plan for their journey before they start while others just jump into their journey and plan later. Still, everyone should have an equal chance to glow, to allow yourself to shine in a way that makes you feel good to be you.

It's my job to bring out the best in every single person I meet. I want those who listen to me to know that I want them to glow as brightly as they possibly can. They may not agree with some of the things I have to say, but then they may not be prepared to glow in the way that they should be. So, it's time to either give up or glow up. To help you with your glow, here are six steps for a glowing mindset:

1. CLEAR YOUR BLOCKAGES

To explain this step clearly, you must see yourself as a manifestation of energy with vibrations. A person can have good energy with good vibes or blocked energy with negative vibes. These vibrations affect the world around you based on how you're feeling; if you've had a good day and are emitting good vibrations, then those vibrations will cause the things around you to look better and the people around you to feel better as well. The opposite is true too, so it's important for you to be aware of the type of energy you're emitting so that you're able to have the best vibrations you can. The art of Reiki is a tool that can be used to help you become more in tune with the vibes that you are emitting and to help them become better for yourself and those around you. When you are physically injured, your first instinct is to put your hand on where you're hurting and attempt to will the pain away. Reiki is similar in this sense, but instead of a physical injury, you're attempting to heal your inner thoughts and vibrations.

To perform Reiki, you need to have a space where you are comfortable sitting or lying down. You don't want any distractions and should be as calm as you can be. You can utilise mediation to help clear your mind or use calming music to focus your thoughts. Next, rub your hands together to focus your energy into your palms. Slowly move your hands along your body, just above the skin, to move your energy. Start at your wrist, then work your way up your arm. You may find your hand staying over one part of your body; this indicates that there's some negative energy in the area or a blockage that you'll need to work through. Allow yourself to focus on where your hands linger, as this will tell you if you're having a problem. Once you've finished working through your body's energy, it's customary to end with touching your feet, known as Grounding. This will allow your focus to become grounded back into the physical world. There's no right or wrong method of focusing on your energies, so take some time to explore a few different methods, to get a better idea as to what works best for you. Know that this will help to align your energy but shouldn't be your main source of healing if you do have a physical condition. Another way to help clear out any negative energy that's made its way into your home is to clean your home. Clear out any items that you don't need any more and clean up any cluttered rooms to make your home more organised. This works as a chance for you to clean your home, but to identify any bad energies that may have found their way into your house and get rid of them. I know after a day of cleaning out my house, I sometimes feel lighter with the accomplishment; this is your glow revealing itself through all the mess and clutter you've worked through.

2. GET ORGANISED

If you've already gone through step one and worked on cleaning your house, it's time to work on organising the things that you still have in your home. Working through your home room by room and making sure that the items in them have a place is imperative for organisation. This step may take some time, depending on the kinds of things you have stored in your rooms. I know first hand that this can take more than just a few days. Working room to room can help you stay on track and pick up where you left off the day before without worry, but there are always going to be hiccups. If you find that you've got a huge number of items that don't have a home yet, leave them and work on another room or another area. Don't get exasperated if you keep finding things that you're not sure you'll be able to use; the key to this step is to sort and organise first and then get rid of anything that doesn't need to be in your home later. If you don't have anything more to throw out or recycle after cleaning a room, that's fine as well.

You don't need to have something to get rid of with every room you organise, since your main task is for sorting. As you go through each room, note if you have too many of a certain item or things that you bought that you never used. Make a mental note that you don't need to go out and buy more, since you don't need them.

This step can also extend to your refrigerator. Prepping for meals is something that's come into the public eye now more than ever and it's a handy tool to make sure that you've got your meals pre-planned if you're on a busy schedule. Organising your meals and shopping so that you can have everything prepared ahead of time not only saves you time but gives you more time to be with your family or friends. Being able to go into your fridge or freezer and pick out something that just needs to be baked or heated up will allow you to have peace of mind and glow with the knowledge that you're sorting has come to fruition.

3. GET STRONGER

So, you've worked through your home and are glowing with the amount of time that you've put in to make sure that negativity doesn't touch you. Now, it's time to focus on getting yourself stronger, both physically and mentally. The food you eat is a huge part of getting yourself stronger. Everyone has their likes and dislikes, so don't try to sacrifice the foods you love just because they aren't considered healthy. The goal is to work with what you're able to eat and prepare them in a way that is best. You don't need to go out and buy superfoods or ingredients that promise a healthier gut; first and foremost, you need to understand what your needs are and how you can fulfil them with the food that you buy.

Start off with what sort of meal plan you're hoping to work through. Speak to your doctor about what types of food they'd recommend you eat more of or avoid to get a baseline. If there is a certain weight goal you're attempting to achieve or part of your health that you want to improve, they are the best resource of information on what you should be eating. Then, you should start going through any recipes or cookbooks that you have and explore cooking websites based on the types of food that your doctor recommended. Any ingredients for those meals that you are missing should go right on your shopping list. If you need to buy vegetables, try to buy them frozen so that they will last longer and can be used for multiple meals. If you're thinking that this whole process might be hard for you to follow, then start small; even the smallest changes can set the foundation for your growth.

Exercising is something that everyone struggles with at some point. There are days when I need to force myself to get out of my warm bed to do my morning exercises. Just like with food, speak to a doctor about what types of exercises would be beneficial for you. In this case, the best way to begin is slowly. Your body may not be used to the kind of workout you're hoping to achieve right away, so you need to train it first. Always stretch before exercising to help minimise any muscle pain; you are going to hurt after a workout, so it's best to help reduce that pain as much as possible. If you hurt yourself during your exercises, don't ever push through it, even if you're determined to finish. Sometimes, something as simple as a sprain can cause problems for you later if you don't take care of it right away. If you don't feel like you're motivated to exercise on your own, a fitness class is a great alternative. You can meet others who are attempting to reach similar goals and your instructor can help motivate you to continue exercising in an environment without judgement. Even going to the gym with a group of friends can help you keep on your routine, as you can help to build each other up and work with one another to reach your fitness goal.

One of the most important things that you'd need to make sure is strong is your mindset. Sure, eating healthy and exercising are all well and good, but if you're not in the right headspace, then you're more likely to not follow what you've planned for your body already. Keeping yourself in a good mood is hard, I won't lie, but knowing what things make you happy and keep yourself feeling positive will assist you in keeping a good mindset. If you find yourself struggling or cannot break yourself out of feelings of doubt or despair, speak with a therapist about the options you have to help improve your mental health. Doing all these steps regularly will get you stronger. This will lead to confidence and with you glowing so bright that you'll feel like you can achieve endless possibilities.

4. GETTING CONFIDENCE

Now that you're working on improving yourself, the next step is to find a concrete goal that you want to work towards. There's so many different things that you can be and the first thing you need to do is focus on exactly what you want to do in life. For most people, this is a tough thing to think about. As we get older, we can become complacent and feel more content with where we are in our lives instead of wishing for a change. You don't want to leave the job you dislike because you'll lose the salary you worked so hard for. You don't want to start up the hobby you want to because you feel like you don't have the time. You don't want to work towards a promotion because you're not confident that you'll get it. All of these thoughts are common, depending on what you want to do. The first step in getting out of these thoughts is to have confidence in yourself. "The worst they can say is no" is a quote that I find myself going back to time and time again. Sure, we may fail if we're trying to get ourselves into a new situation, but the point is to not stop and to keep trying. If you don't like your job, put in the work to search for one that will give you exactly what you're hoping for in a position. If you want to start a new hobby, make the time to try it out and see if it's something that you want to keep doing. If you want to go for a promotion, show your boss that you're interested and have the skills for it. The worst thing that could happen is that you're rejected and need to rethink your way of approaching the situation. Try another method, rework your strategy, don't allow yourself to be complacent. Be confident in your abilities. Glow with the desire for your true self, the person that you really are, and you'll find that so many doors will open for you.

5. DECISION MAKING

All the desires of your new life will mean nothing if you don't actually make clear decisions. You can wish and dream about the life you want to live, but if you don't have a clear plan and decision for what your life is going to be like, then all of the work you put into your idea of a new life will remain just that, an idea. And even if you begin to work towards the decision you make, there shouldn't be any reason for you to abruptly stop.

There are so many people out in the world with amazing ideas for things as small as how they're going to decorate their room to how to plan their wedding. They come up with these amazing plans and vision boards to help them focus on what would be best. Then, after a few weeks of having that board up, they toss it and start another one. The cycle repeats until they're forced into a decision that wasn't a part of their plan at all. The last thing you want to do is not give yourself the opportunity to make your own decisions on how you're going to move with your life. Understand the kind of work that would go into a decision and know exactly what you want before you begin your planning. This will help you to focus and be able to make the decision you want without any compromises.

6. TAKE ACTION

You can have all your ducks in a row but if you don't put all your inner and outer glowing work that you have done so far into action, then nothing will happen. Actually going out and making the things you dreamed about a reality is hard work and requires you to remain focused on your goals and aspirations. However, perseverance is key to make sure that the actions you take for your new life are fulfilled and done to the best of their ability.

Have you ever had a feeling of excitement come over you, like you could feel something was about to happen? That is the universe saying it's here, come and get it. Take glowing action or the unseen opportunity will pass you by. Don’t just wait for yourself to glow, get yourself glowing now so that you can become the person you truly want to be.

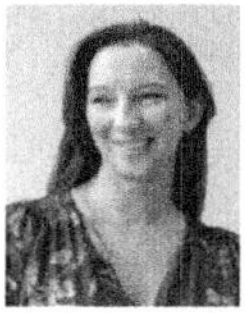

About Rebecca Landy

Rebecca Landy is the founder of "GLOW LIFE & STYLE".

She is a Personal Glowing Transformational Coach for women, it is her quest to help as many women GLOW their best in all things mind body and soul, she will help you achieve a GLOW in all aspects of life just with a bit of Style thrown in!!!

As a trained Dancer and Fitness Instructor, Reiki Master, Meditation Facilitator and Beauty Consultant Specialising in Luxury Tanning Experiences, particularly Bridal Tans and her Training for Self Reiki and Spray Tan Business Mentorship in her Glow Training Academy she is known for her Courses, Workshops and Luxury Events and Retreats.

Rebecca's Goal and purpose is to provide not just high quality Services or Trainings but to do so with the purpose of increase - wanting all woman to have an "Experience" which leaves you with more than you expected and wanting more because you have been awakened to more...

Who is this for??

Women who either want to find their Glow or have a burning desire to rekindle a Glow they once had but lost it somewhere along the way. Rebecca will take you on a journey of self-discovery, clear any negative energy blocks helping to create a Self Image you can be proud of and eliminating old beliefs that hold you back. Rebecca will help you set new goals in life to create the glowing life and style you wish to lead.

If you want an inner and outer Glow that radiates confidence, strength and well-being then Rebecca is the GLOWING Coach for you. Join her in person or online for any of her Classes, Events, Workshops or Special Luxury Retreats or if you want to train with her then the Academy is for you, whatever way you wish to work with Rebecca she will get you GLOWING in Life & Style.

Connect with Rebecca at:

- Landyrebecca@hotmail.com
- https://www.facebook.com/GLOW-LIFE-STYLE-DanceFit-ness-Beauty-Holistic-Wellness-120284663174209/

Movement Is Medicine

By Adele Smyth

"The Mind when housed in a healthful body possesses a glorious sense of power." Joseph Pilates

I've always been a bit of a performer and like being in front of an audience. I've always wanted to share my love of how good moving your body and exercising can make you feel. I try not to show off, but at the same time, I won't shy away from being in the spotlight. I think it must be in my genes. My Uncle was the All-Ireland Irish dance champion when he was younger, and my Dad was on 'Come Dancing' on TV before it became 'Strictly'! Dancing seems to have always been in my blood and in my soul.

Countless ballet shoes and pointe shoes now exist in my closets and attic as wonderful memories of my childhood and my years of dancing. I'm thrilled that my passion for dance and movement as a child has seen me through my journey to where I am now. That it has supported me through times of sorrow and through life disruptions. Exercise and movement have fuelled my passion to enable me to pass on my experiences, knowledge and skills to others, to make them start to like themselves again and to feel good in their own skin.

I began dancing when I was around 5 years old. It started with the obligatory children's ballet and tap classes and then, as I grew older, it became an integral part of me. I danced my way through school, college, and university. I found that dancing was something that came naturally and I enjoyed it, even when I was participating in competitions. As I grew older, I shied away from more traditional ballet and began to work on a style that was my own.

When I was in my early 30's we lost my Dad to cancer. Dancing became a way for me to focus on something other than my grief. Looking back on that time, I utilised my dancing as a form of therapy, even if I didn't realise it at the time. My dancing became a way for me to stay healthy and to work my body when my mind was full, which in turn, helped to empty my mind and allowed my jumbled thoughts to become organised. As the years went by, I found myself turning to physical exercise as a way to get out of my head if I was stressed or overwhelmed.

Exercise and physical fitness have definitely saved me numerous times over the years. It has kept me sane when having to juggle two jobs to keep a roof over my children's heads and food on the table. As a single mother, there were times when I worried about where our next meal was coming from, but my determination in keeping my mind and body strong kept my thoughts unclouded as I found my niche as a fitness instructor. However, the thing that has saved me the most has been my 'Why?'. What is a 'Why?' A 'Why' is the reason you get out of bed every morning. A 'Why' is something that you know you can't ever live without, or you'll lose all motivation. A 'Why' can be a person, an event, a goal that's within your reach. For me, my 'Why' describes my daughters. They are the reason that even when I was exhausted from working a shift as a nurse, I would come home and, after giving them dinner, we would all go to the local village hall so I could teach my classes. I'd be able to work through my tiredness in order to make sure that I could show them that I was doing something that I enjoyed and not just making money.

I learned a lot through my time as a Pilates instructor and I'd like to think it helped me to understand things about others a bit more. Working with other people and helping them to exercise in a way that they probably weren't familiar with showed me how to be open and understanding. Some of my students couldn't stretch very far or were unsure as to how to get their bodies in certain positions. I admit, at the start, I had to stop myself from being annoyed at the students that needed more attention. Now, I welcome it, as I know that they're doing their best and have come to my class to get my assistance with their minds and bodies. Whichever stage of life or circumstance you're in, one thing will always remain equally important: good health, both physical and emotional. A strong body can help to support a strong mind and a strong mind helps to provide for a strong body. Just like anything else, we achieve this stability in different ways because we are different people. I wanted to find a space that would allow me to nurture others' thoughts on this and help them to develop themselves in ways they didn't think they could. Creating a safe space for my clients and a place to enjoy movement and fitness led me to create Purebody by Adele and develop The Purebody Technique over 16 years ago. This has been a labour of love, a wonderful experience and a firm goal to of mine is to make others feel good about themselves again. To celebrate how amazing our body can be and to know that we are doing the best we can for ourselves. The goal of my class is to help you to be the best body for the body that you have, and for you to be able to achieve this through movement, health and wellness. It's a labour of love that I've hoped has helped those that have made their way into my class.

I'm open with my clients about how important I think it is to say if you're not ok when someone asks how you are, and that it is ok not to be ok. There's something to be said about the world today, where our responses to stress and adversity is to try and tamp our own emotions down. We should be able to express ourselves without the norm of society telling us that it's not okay to be so emotional. I've found, both through internal investigation and through talking with my students, that it's the element of control that helps us ground ourselves when things get to be too much.

Of course, we can't control every situation that we come across, that's not possible, unfortunately. However, establishing a routine as a way to give yourself something to look forward to after a long day of work can do wonders in helping to keep your mind as sound as you want your body to be. I make sure to ask these questions to my clients to have them focus on certain things while in my classesand I make sure to reflect on them myself to get a better perspective on my own life. With these questions, I hope to get myself and others thinking about how they're proceeding with their routines and if there's anything they want to change:

- How often do you put yourself first?
- Do you ever put your mental health first or focus solely on your physical health?
- Would you chat with someone about how you truly feel, or do you feel that being honest could be a burden on them and they may not understand?

Making goals that are realistic and achievable is the key to how we get to the place we want to be, both physically and mentally. When it comes to our health and fitness, why do we assume that if we haven't seen an immediate change in ourselves that we are failing? We are all built differently and respond to life stresses and strains, both environmental and physical, in different ways. Don't just assume that something isn't working for you because you don't see immediate results, but don't push yourself to continue with a routine that you don't believe is a good fit for you. This is the same for mental health as well. You can't expect your mental health to improve after just a few days of a new routine. It's all about keeping up with that routine so that you'll be able to see the results.

It took me a long time to appreciate how athletic and strong my body was and continues to be. I look back on how long it took me to give myself permission to like the athletic build that I had and not concern myself with trying to transform my body into something it wasn't.

I want to provide you with that same kind of acceptance that I learned to give myself. I want you to be able to look at yourself and know that you're improving your body and mind, even if the changes don't seem substantial at the time. I want you to be able to utilise exercise in a way that can give you the strength you need when other methods don't seem viable.

There's a very common saying that "Rome wasn't built in a day." In the same way, our bodies and minds are not built overnight either. We can't just set a goal for ourselves, then throw out that goal if we aren't seeing results as quickly as we wanted to. The key is to take things day by day and not focus on the goal as a permanent endgame. You will need to be flexible with your goals so that you can show yourself that you can reach them. Don't give yourself a set timeline; instead, focus on the little changes you can make that will work you up to your main goal for your body and mind.

I like to tell my students that if they have an endgame goal, they should sit down and break that goal down to its barest parts in order to find out what they can do to achieve it. For example, if you want to work on losing weight, you'd need to set a goal for how much weight you want to lose. From there, it's looking at your current life and routine and finding ways to either cut out unhealthy habits or create healthy habits. You might find that you have an extra snack shortly after breakfast to give yourself a boost of energy while you're at work; you may not want to get rid of that snack because it helps keep you focused at the beginning of your day. Instead of cutting it out completely, you may want to substitute your usual snack with something healthier. It's little changes that can add up and help make whatever goal you have not seem as daunting.

You're not alone in thoughts of frustration and intimidation when it comes to reaching your health goal. It's safe to say that we've all been there at some point. And there can be points where you feel like you'll need to give up on that goal because you're not seeing any progress or you've fallen back onto habits you were hoping to avoid. I'm here to tell you that it's okay if you've reached that point. We are not perfect and running into roadblocks on our way to our goals isn't uncommon. The key is to find ways to overcome those blocks.

I found that the best way to assist with those roadblocks is to surround yourself with those who are willing to lift you up and support your goals. I want my classes to be a place that my students feel supported in, no matter what goal they have in mind, so I try to keep negativity to a minimum. They can work together to lift each other up without judgement and maybe teach each other ways to help get to their goals. In the end, I know I've done my job when one of my students reaches a smaller goal and is met with cheers of support from their classmates.

We all have the ability to hold onto a realistic end result and a desire to feel and be what we want. To know that we can have a functionally fit and healthy body which will remain strong for us to be able to continue to perform all activities of our daily life. For me this desire should never fade or be dismissed. Within us I believe we all have the fire and drive to push ourselves forward to continue to move towards our ultimate goal and to tell ourselves to never give up.

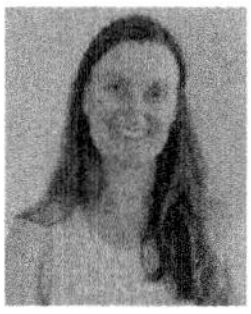

About Adele Smyth

Adele helps women to regain their body confidence and strength following changes to their body that they may have experienced during their life. Using her bespoke Purebody Method which incorporates elements of Pilates, Ballet, Yoga and Women's Health, Adele helps to heal dysfunction within our body that may have arisen over the years. Adele's method and teaching will improve muscle balance and overall body performance; enabling you to remain active and live with ease as you move through your life's chapters.

As a Pilates and Yoga teacher, as well as a women's health specialist, Adele has been involved in the health and wellness industry for over 25 years. Adele's interest in health and fitness began at the age of 3 when she started ballet and contemporary dance classes. Adele's passion for dance and movement continued into her teens and beyond and led her to train as a fitness instructor in her 20's and later as a Pilates, Yoga and BalletBeFit teacher.

As a registered nurse Adele has extensive medical knowledge and utilises this within her teaching and her Purebody Method. Rather than focusing purely on aesthetics as a goal, Adele is keen to encourage women to become more aware of the strength within their body and their mind, and to remind themselves of how amazing their bodies are in supporting us day in and day out. The added element of women's health has helped many women to continue to live a normal life without the fear that they will have pelvic floor dysfunction.

Adele has a holistic, full body approach to health and wellness and has recognised that using massage therapy as part of her Method will improve the outcomes that women are striving to achieve, as it is important to lengthen a muscle and release areas of tightness before we strengthen and tone our body. Reduced muscle movement prevents our body moving to its full range and can be a cause of discomfort and pain. Adele's bespoke Method will highlight specific areas which need attention and work to improve these.

With injury prevention in mind, Adele focuses on safety in her classes and how to progress movements to ensure that your body is warm and prepared to move. Adele firmly believes that connecting to your body via movement leaves you feeling joyful and energised and loves watching women transform themselves from feeling disconnected from their body to being proud of who they are.

Connect with Adele at:

- adele@purebodybyadele.co.uk
- www.purebodybyadele.co.uk

Follow Your Dream

By Daniela Berei

Just because you are an adult doesn't mean you have to give up your unfulfilled childhood dreams.

My childhood dream was to do ballet. I loved dancing to my favourite songs and I was always very graceful. I don't know where my love for ballet started, but I know that it has followed me all my life. I would watch ballet on the television and the dancers seemed like the most graceful beings in the world. I adored them and dreamt that one day, I would be like them; gracefully dancing and leaping through the air with such poise. The way that they moved their hands and fingers while dancing fascinated me, and I wondered how someone could be so graceful as to control their bodies up to their fingertips. My parents enrolled me in a popular art school in Romania where I studied the violin, ballet, and aerobic gymnastics. I was fascinated by ballet and my interest in dancing became a major focus for me. However, the school didn't have a special ballet class and my aerobic gymnastics took precedence, but nothing made me give up on my dream. I remember how we started our lessons at the barre in gymnast costumes. The years passed and my fascination for ballet did not leave me for a second.

Why has ballet remained in my mind and my soul? Because, through ballet, I felt that I could fly into a parallel world, one with a different way of breathing, a release of emotions that I'd never felt, a poem I could perform as a dance.

However, because I didn't follow it while in school, it remained like a small flame that did not go out of my mind and my soul. It was ever present within me, but I didn't allow it to grow as much as it could have. It was always on my mind that I would be able to do ballet. When I was young, I would close my eyes and think of something beautiful that I wanted to happen for me. I would envision myself floating through an azure sky full of music, grace, and emotion, my dancing able to take me off the ground. I felt like I had a connection to soft music with the rhythm of great composers behind it. I felt that ballet was the way for me to explore beauty and cultivate my spirit. Ballet for me was not only a form of artistic expression, but also exemplified happiness and relaxation to have me be more in touch with my emotions.

My love for ballet and the dream in my mind to dance helped to raise my self-esteem through strength, control, and discipline. I knew these to be the foundation of ballet and even though I wasn't able to dance, I still wanted to rework those virtues into my line of work as I grew older. I began a career as a nurse and found that the two had much in common. Working as a nurse, my job relies heavily on my communication with others in my field. I need to be alert and ready to take action, leaping, in a way, to make sure that my patients are receiving their best care. I learned to watch how my patients moved and how to work with them to get where we needed to go. I began to watch my own body for signs of fatigue or burnout so that someone else could continue the routine I set and I could rest and recuperate.

Outside of work, I continued with exercises at home in order to stay fit. I tried the gym, weight training, and cardio, but I didn't find myself truly enjoying any of them. They felt like just another addition to my routine and lacked the grace that I was looking for. A part of me wanted to find a class that focused on ballet techniques, but I was too afraid. I was over forty and there was no way that I could still follow that dream of mine without failing miserably after so long.

A Chance to Dream

A few months ago, I met Rachel Withers at an online event for the "BBF 5 Day Challenge." The event encouraged me to follow my dream, even though I was over forty, to do a ballet fitness class. Rachel explained step by step on how I could make a business out of my dream. She encouraged me to do what I wanted and that it's never too late to fulfil your dream. She told me about a fifty-year-old woman who did ballet. The woman was just as hesitant as I was, but she wanted to fulfil her dream. Rachel said that the woman didn't have the opportunity as a child, as she got married young and the obligations of married life became her priority. The woman finally had the time to focus on her dreams after years and years of focusing on other things. Rachel taught me through that story and her teachings that it is important to live your dream anytime at any age. She told me that one day, I'd meet a person or people that would resonate with my passion for ballet and could inspire me to try it. I just needed to be open to those encounters. My dream came true after I passed the age of forty. I know that I will not be the greatest ballerina of all time, but that is not my goal. I finally gave myself the opportunity to take a class that I had avoided because I thought I was too old. In addition, there are benefits that ballet exercises could provide me that would make sure I was limber and graceful as I could be. It's a fantastic way to keep fit and to develop and maintain flexibility. To me, ballet meant strength, concentration, self-discipline, mobility, balance, elegance, and grace. I didn't think I'd be able to still achieve these virtues in my older age, but I did and I still am reaping their benefits.

The Art of the Dream

Ballet has inspired people who perceive it as something from a scene in a movie; when the protagonist breaks into a dance to escape from everyday problems and forget about the stress of their lives. This beautiful art that is ballet has been considered more than a sport and allows practitioners to achieve a body with harmonious development. It's not something that someone can master through their first class, but comes with practice and training over time. No matter how hard it was to reach my dream as an adult, the satisfaction of my success is enormous; it's not something that can be explained in words, but through feelings.

I still have much to learn, but I am persistent and I will not give up. The online classes with Rachel Withers are a balm for my soul and my body. The most important thing that I discovered was that I can still achieve the grace I was looking to have when I was a young girl and nothing can stop me from fulfilling my childhood dream of doing ballet.

Fulfilling Your Dream

I don't know what dreams you each have, but I know you should never give them up. Your age or people's comments should not stop you from fulfilling your dream. Happiness is a thing that gives each person the courage and freedom to live life the way they want. If you feel this is something that you're ready for, take a deep breath and turn your passion into reality. Passion is a force that can literally move mountains. Passion is the engine of social and personal evolution. I learned that through my ballet classes as the flame in my heart began to burn brighter and brighter with my passion for dancing. I am able to fly, to run, to bend and bow. I can do all these things as long as I dream. In order to fulfil your dream you need to study and work to evolve. To dream means to dive into your thoughts and discover who you really are. I am currently living my dream of ballet and I love that I can fulfil the dream I had for myself so many years ago. Whether it is a word or an image, a dream must be shaped. The next step is to put it on paper or keep it in our mind focused and carry it with us so that you always remember your dream. From this moment, you'll know that you are one step closer to the moment when it will be fulfilled. While focusing on my dream, I read the works of Jacques Salome. He was a famous French psychologist and the initiator of the Hope method, which he utilises in order to have a specific desire fulfilled. There are whole articles and books on this, but I will highlight a few guidelines.

First, desire nourishes the dream. Build your project well so that you know your limits. Describe the steps you have to go through in order to get where you wish to be. Success is achieved by desire! So long as you have passion for your dream, you cannot go wrong.

Dreaming and Desires

I am on the verge of realising my childhood dream because I met Rachel, who instilled in me the courage I needed and urged me to fulfil my dream of ballet. All of us need that reminder that there are people who believe in us, regardless of our age, and who wish to support us in achieving our dreams. I believe that we must help our children, from an early age, to try to fulfil their dreams and offer them the necessary tools to help them. Your time has come. It is time to go your own way, do what you love, give up being unhappy. Don't wait for tomorrow, not when you have more time, or when you will retire. Today is the day!

Today is the day when your dream begins to come true, when there is no fear and everything is possible. Have you ever wondered what you have done so far for your dream? Did you have the motivation to go ahead and evolve to fulfil your dream?

Albert Einstein once said that, "The mind is like a parachute. It works well only when it is open."

We need to dream and have goals. We need to be alert and ready for those dreams to be fulfilled so that we don't become complacent in our lives, and we aren't constantly asking ourselves what we should be doing. The worst thing you can do is to keep your dream in your soul, to hide it only for yourself because you didn't have the courage to take it out for the world to see. You might not have the courage to give it colour or never do anything to nourish and feed the flame inside of you. A hidden dream that remains inside can become a regret and it can hurt you the longer you keep it locked away and unfulfilled. A dream is a desire of the soul and the soul always speaks; we just need to listen to it. Napoleon Hill said that, "Anything that the mind can think and the heart can love, you can accomplish." In other words, there are no impossible dreams, so long as you have that dream and it was realised by you. This requires courage, determination and desire.

How? If you're having trouble realising your dream, focus on this question to help you:

If you had all the resources in the world, be it time, money, health, friends, and family, what would you do?

This question helps you detach yourself from the limits of autonomy and allows your soul to express itself without limits. The answer that will come from within will show you what you really want. Without limitations, you can find a way to make a plan to get there. You need a plan because you have to imagine that your dream is already fulfilled. This will help you to envision what you want for your dream and how you hope to achieve it.

It is said that every person comes to earth with a talent. We all have skills unique to us, even if we may not realise them right away. Somehow, when we are young, we do what we must do and grow believing that other things are a priority to our thoughts and dreams. If we're not careful, we can deprive our soul of our dreams and live out our lives half fulfilled.

How do we know that we will cope with what we dreamed? The best answer comes from Marianne Williamson: "Our biggest fear is not that we are inadequate but that we are too strong. Our light and not the darkness within us frightens us the most. We often wonder who I am to be bright, wonderful, talented, fabulous? There is nothing great about shrinking yourself so that others do not feel insecure with you. We are all meant to shine, and this is not in only some of us but in each person. When we let our own light shine, we give others permission to do the same. When we free ourselves from our own fear, our presence automatically frees others."

When you meet a person who is living out their dream, there are probably a few questions that you have:

- How did it all start?
- How did you know what you wanted to do?
- Did you have any talents to help you?
- Was it hard for you?
- How dare you?

We may fixate on others who we see as obstacles in

fulfilling our dreams or think that they see themselves as better than us because they're already doing what they love. We need to focus on ourselves and realise that everyone achieves their dreams at their own pace. It's not a race to see who can fulfil their dream first.

I've found that the biggest obstacles in fulfilling a dream are:

- Social programming
- Limited beliefs
- Fear
- Lack of know-how
- Lack of recourse

Setting a goal or defining a dream should be done as something measurable and without attempting to compare it to someone else. If it is your dream, surely something in you pushes you forward, even if you are in a difficult situation. Remind yourself of the reasons why you wanted your dream. Are those reasons still valid or have they changed over time? Ask yourself how your life will change after you have fulfilled your dream or goal. That perspective should motivate you. If not, you should look to open the parachute. Remember that if you have been given a dream, it means that you can make it come true. It only depends on you.

So what happens when we believe in our dream but others don't? When no one believes in our dream, we close our ears to the criticism, and seek to encourage ourselves with people who support us. Is it good to talk about your dreams? That was always a very important question to me, so I will provide you with the answers I found, my dear reader. If the person you tell about your dream is a friend or a person who supports you and encourages you unconditionally, then you've shared it with the right person.

If the person you speak to does not believe in you or sees only the negative side of things, then this person will not be able to help you reach your dream and may even hinder you.

Too Late to Fulfil a Dream?

There is no set time limit for a dream. It is never too late to start doing something you have always wanted to do. No matter your age, you can work on your dream and allow it to fuel your passion. You can feel an unseen force carrying you to your dream. When the dream becomes strong enough, it can provide you with all the strength and courage you need.. I am proof that it is never too late to fulfil your dream. My dream and my attitude about my dream gave me the results I wanted. I had a dream and that meant a goal that I set in order to achieve it. I am an ambitious person and I strongly believe in my dream even after it's been fulfilled. Over time, I realised that I needed a lot of patience. A part of me believed that if I didn't manage to see my dream fulfilled as a child, I'd never see it brought to life. Now, as an adult, I was able to do what I needed to in order to fulfil my dream. I enjoy the freedom and the beautiful people and things that surround me and build me up to reach my dream. To dream means to immerse yourself in your thoughts and discover who you really are. Sometimes these dreams seem difficult or impossible to fulfil and even though you want them to become a reality, you may not have the motivation and strength to follow them. Because your dreams are part of your soul, they will remain there and will only provide you with true happiness if you give them life.

With that in mind, I've prepared a collection of my favourite motivational quotes. These sayings have helped me through my life and I hope that they will resonate with you as well.

- "All our dreams can come true if we have the courage to follow them." **-Walt Disney**
- "Nothing great in the world has been accomplished without passion." **-George Wilhelm**
- "Once you choose hope, anything is possible."- **Christopher Reeve**
- "I think one of the biggest risks in life is to never have the courage to take a risk." **-Oprah Winfrey**
- "If you don't risk it, you will never be defeated. But you will never win either." **-Richard Nixon**
- "You must constantly try to climb very high if you want to be able to see very far." **-Constantin Brancusi**
- "Keep your dreams to yourself! If dreams die, life becomes a bird with broken wings which cannot fly." - **Langston Hughes**
- "Appreciate your vision and dreams, because they are the children of your soul: the sketches of your supreme achievements." **-Napoleon Hill**

- "Don't put limits on anything. The more you dream, the further you go." **-Michael Phelps**
- "It is the mark of an inexperienced man not to believe in luck." **-Conrad**
- "A dream does not become reality through magic: it takes sweat, determination, and hard work." - **Colin Powell**
- "If you think you can't, you are right .If you think you can, you are right again." **-Henry Ford**
- "Get to work with all your heart and you will succeed. The competition is so small." **-Elbert Hubbard**
- "Don't get pushed into matters. Let yourself be driven by dreams." **-Ralph Waldo Emerson**.
- "Fly to the moon. Even if you don't succeed, at least you will be among the stars." **-Lee Brown**
- "All the dreaming in the world will not matter if you are not ready to wake up and get to work."- **John C. Maxwell**
- "When you want something, all the universe conspires in helping you to achieve it." **-Pablo Coelho**.
- "Miracles happen to those who believe in them." - **Bernhard Berenson**
- "If you do not think about the future, you cannot have one." **-Galsworthy**
- "It is a happiness to wonder, it is a happiness to dream." **-Edgar Alan Poe**
- "The best revenge is massive success." **-Frank Sinatra**
- "The best way to predict the future is to create it." - **Peter Drucker**
- "Logic will get from A to B. Imagination will take you anywhere." **-Albert Einstein**

- "Nothing is impossible for the one who tries." - **Alexandru Macedon**
- "Life is like riding a bicycle. To keep your balance, you must keep moving." -**Albert Einstein**
- "Success is the ability to go from failure without losing your enthusiasm." -**Winston Churchill**
- "Happiness is when you think, what you say, and what you do are in harmony." -**Mahatma Gandhi**.
- "There are only two ways to live your life. One is as though nothing is a miracle. The other is as though everything is a miracle." -**Albert Einstein**
- "Everything you can imagine is real." -**Pablo Picasso**
- "Go confidently in the direction of your dreams. Live the life you have imagined." -**Ralph Waldo Emerson**
- "Keep love in your heart. A life without it is like a sunless garden when the flowers are dead." - **Oscar Wilde**
- "Choose a job you love, and you will never have to work a day in your life." -**Confucius**
- "In the middle of difficulty lies opportunity." - **Albert Einstein**
- "I never dreamed about success. I worked for it." - **Estee Lauder**
- "Accept responsibility for your life. Know that it is you who will get you where you want to go, no one else." -**Les Brown**

Every dream is like a flame that burns slowly in our soul until we decide to give it oxygen to grow. Every dream has a story that can be turned into a successful book!

Let your dream guide you in your life.

So what are you waiting for? Follow your dream!

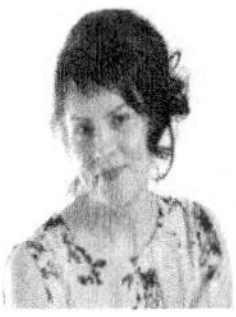

About Daniela Berei

Daniela is from Romania and has been a nurse for twenty years. Her specialty is an Adult General Nurse.

In 1995 she started working at: Radio, TV in her city of Calarasi and also for the local newspaper. She was very successful and was encouraged to continue on this path of journalism, however she chose the profession of being a nurse. She felt that she could give more of her kindness to treat the patients.

Communication and empathy have been key to her success because with the job comes both physical and emotional challenges, finding balance between stress and peaceful days, tears and smiling, hold hands till the end ...and memories. Since 1997 until 2000, Daniela followed the course of sanitary Post-Secondary School in Calarasi. The three years of study were one of the most beautiful years of her life, in which prepared her to work as a general nurse. Daniela has realised that the nursing profession is associated with a tremendous amount of satisfaction, rewards, opportunities, and challenges.

From the teacher and doctors' stories Daniela identified several things which inspired and motived her to work as a nurse. The most important thing was that she could help those who suffer. Every day for twenty years each day has been a special day with achievements, tears, and soul satisfactions and both beautiful and annoying experiences, but all of them contribute to the woman she is today. She has shared experiences with special medical staff who motivated her, and patients that she will never forget. This has led her to the understanding that her role is not just taking care of patients from the medical point of view, but also that she spends time with them and helps them to relieve their pain. In addition to medical care the nurse meets the emotional, social and spiritual needs of the patients, having the possibility to treat the patient as a whole person, body and soul. In other words, we become their angels.

In the year 2000 Daniela became an adult general nurse and has worked in both the private and the public health system offering quality medical care to patients. Daniela believes when you choose this profession, you assume to be present in any situation, whether that's positive, when everything is productive, when the patient feels well and there is a pleasant and satisfying atmosphere to when everything seems to be collapsing. The job needs a balance of professionalism and humanity.

Daniela has learnt from her experience as a nurse to appreciate simply living her life beyond measure and every moment has to be savoured and treasured. Throughout these years Daniela hasn't forgotten her dream: to do Ballet everyday. Modesty, Grace and Courage helped Daniela to become a nurse but also to follow her dream and dance.

Connect with Daniela at:

- daniela.berei@balletbefit.com

Embracing Change with Loving Eyes and a Grateful Heart

By Nancy Cashman

Change is inevitable. It's a constant that affects everything from the smallest action to the biggest. It ebbs and flows throughout the tapestries of our lives without reason and without warning. We can go through a routine that we have set one day and then the next have that routine change because of an unforeseen event. All change brings about a new set of circumstances, in its own way, regardless of whether that change is "good" or "bad."

For instance, an engagement is a "happy" change, but it presents the challenge of bringing two families together harmoniously. This too brings on its own changes and with it, challenges: where will the family live, how many children and/or pets do they see themselves having, at whose parents' house do they spend the holidays, and similar questions. These changes can be exciting, yet there are still unknown factors that will arise, along with compromises and concessions that need to be made to make the changes successful ones. Other changes that deal with health issues and getting older may seem to fall on the spectrum of "sad" or "bad" changes, but there are ways to see those changes as good. We can remain true to ourselves as our bodies age and to celebrate where we've been through and how far we've come. We need to embrace the now, and the change that comes with that to accompany us along for the journey, without getting caught up in the limitations imposed by society and culture.

Limitations brought on by changes are inevitable. Yes, there are many legitimate circumstances that do have limitations, it's the nature of the beast, and that's part of life. I'm referring not only to the limitations that we allow others to project onto us, but also to those limitations that we bring upon ourselves. We might be told that we're too old to do something or to act our age. We might have an illness and it has slowed us down or made us not as agile and flexible as we once were. We might be embarrassed with how many wrinkles we have or how our bodies have shifted. We might wonder with our ever-evolving figure, how could we ever wear workout clothes again. Recognizing that limitations are a part of the changes in our lives is the first step in overcoming them and embracing change as a force of nature that can be a positive for you.

When I think of the changes in my life and the limitations that have come with it, I often reflect on two words: Prison and Prism. What is the connection of these two words besides both starting with a "P" and consisting of two syllables? To me, these two words are as connected as opposite sides of the spectrum. When we have limiting beliefs surrounding ourselves and swirling in our heads, it creates a kind of prison in our minds. We're not going to try new things or explore different places because we're locked into a mindset that won't allow us to. However, if we embrace the changes in our lives and see through the limitations that accompany them, we can see our situations in a different light. Our lives, our circumstances, and our surroundings – much like a prism can change your view as you look at it from different angles, so too can we see the more positive sides of our changes along with the brilliant colors it can present.

I've suffered from migraines since I was four years old. The pain was excruciating, and I learned to make my way through life avoiding situations that would bring the migraines on. When I was in my early thirties, I was practically bedridden with fibromyalgia for a year in a time prior to it becoming a recognized condition. My doctors were unsure of what was truly wrong with me and could only provide so much insight without being completely sure as to what I had. I remember being given many different medicines to assist with my conditions and help to provide me some relief.

However, it was a catch-22; I needed sleep and exercise to help negate the symptoms of my migraines, yet there were many times I was in such pain that I couldn't move or sleep. I was told that the body repairs itself during sleep, so when I didn't get any, I knew that my body wasn't healing from whatever sickness I had. I went from doctor to doctor, trying to get some sense into what could be wrong with me and get some sort of relief my symptoms.

I could hardly hold a cup of coffee. It was a rough time in my life and there were points where I wondered if I'd ever get my life back as I knew it.

After being taken to yet another physician and prescribed some additional pain medication and muscle relaxer, I was told that I should join a support group for people with chronic pain to help with coping with my condition. It was after that referral that I had an "aha moment." I took time to reflect on the changes going on in my life and the limitations that came with it and I saw things in a different light. A path forward emerged, and I told myself with certainty that I refused to let this condition control me any longer; I was going to control it! It had taken so much from me already.

I began, with my family doing what they could to support me, to get back to ice skating, dance and high impact aerobics (in which I was certified to teach). They were activities that I loved doing earlier on in my life and that brought me joy, but my condition made me stop because they were too much on my body. I slowly began to ease myself back into those activities, my family encouraging me as best they could. Bit by bit, my body started to get stronger. It took months and months of physical work, but I finally started to feel like myself again. It was a blessing that I am thankful for every day since.

Have my headaches or pain ever totally gone away? No. Some days, it's very hard to get up and keep going through the day, but I push through it as best as I can. In embracing the change and seeing through the prism of my limitation,

I had made a new heartfelt agreement with my body and my soul. I was not going to take my life for granted. I would appreciate where I was at each given moment, living in the now, and be thankful that I had the ability to use it in simple ways that others might not. I didn't measure my progress from how high I used to lift my leg until now or that I could do splits when I wasn't in constant pain. I might never get back to how my body was in its prime, but I've accepted that reality. I need to accept where I am at this very moment.

One of my mantras is, "Be Here, Be Now." This affirmation has allowed me to embrace every milestone as I get stronger. I still convey this mantra and way of thinking to each class or client I teach; I've made sure that it's clear to my students to be grateful, thankful, and appreciative of what you have each and every day. We can't live in the past, no matter how good or glamorous our pasts were. We need to assess and accept where our bodies are at each moment in time and, in turn, that will help us to get stronger and celebrate and embrace every milestone of what we're able to do. I tell my students not to focus on the limitations – look through them for a path forward to wellness in body and spirit. I make sure to let them know that they don't have to be afraid of the limitations either, as they are an inevitable part of the changes that everyone goes through. It's how you adapt to change and how you work through your limitations that makes all the difference, and that can lead you to a better and more peaceful place

Through my migraines and fibromyalgia, there was only so much I was able to do at the beginning of my recovery, I did a lot of visualization along with celebrating each milestone no matter how small. I was introduced to Kundalini Yoga almost four years ago. One of the very insightful lessons of Kundalini Yoga is that, if you can't do an exercise, you should visualize yourself doing it and going through the motions and emotions of it. The benefits are almost the same as actually physically performing the exercise. It gives your mind the practice of focusing on an action and letting the emotions that come with that action affect you. These exercises provide a visualization for all, in order to focus on it as not just an exercise that can be performed without pain, but as a way to see what we could be capable of once our bodies gained more strength. Once I worked through my doubts and began appreciating and being grateful for whatever my body was able to do, I realized the mind and body connection in a different light. I had broken out of the prison and was seeing my life, body and soul, through a new prism.

I have always loved music and movement; it's been a part of my entire life and is such an integral part of my being. At the beginning of my acceptance process, and with my body on the mend after so much inactivity, I was trying a lot of things I had done before. I was easily discouraged by the fact that my body grew tired or hurt more after I had a dance session or went on the ice. I began looking to other activities that I loved, I had done yoga for years and loved how relaxed it could make my body and mind. I decided to take yoga teacher training, not so much as a way for me to learn how to teach, but to get a deeper understanding of the philosophy and the poses.

I was out of my comfort zone in my training classes; I was either the oldest or second oldest person in the training. It didn't matter, I was embraced by the other students. We were required to teach both a class to our fellow students along with a separate community class in our training to qualify for our certification. I was so nervous, but something happened while I was in front of my fellow students leading the class for the first time. I felt transformed by the magic of being able to help and guide people to a relaxing and calming state through my knowledge and care. I started out nervous and within a couple of minutes it became not about me but about giving to others, I was leading from my heart and my fellow yogis were accepting and receptive. I felt such an inner peace that I hadn't expected.

After teaching the community class, a lovely woman I had never met before stopped to tell me that it was the best yoga class she had ever taken. She'd been to many classes at the center and the teachers were all wonderful, I know this for a fact, since I had taken all of their classes many times along with having to write my observations of several classes for my training. My class touched her; she could tell that I wanted to teach the class what I knew and that I was happy to be doing it. Even if she had said this just to be kind, it gave me the belief that I really would be able to do it. This newfound confidence helped me to study for and obtain other certifications in Meditation,

Reiki and BalletBeFit, not to mention establish my own wellness and yoga training company.

Just recently, after almost nine years, I was finally able to thank Hope, the woman who had faith in me along with the kindness she showed by taking a moment to show her gratitude. Had it not been for her words at that moment, who knows if I would have ever taken that first step. I can't even imagine where I would be now if not for her words. I was out of my comfort zone in a world I hadn't fully realized my potential in, yet I embraced the change, saw a path forward through the limitations, and proved my limiting beliefs were wrong. And I can say with all certainty that you can too!

I enjoy working with all clients, but my passion is for helping those who are dealing with serious health issues, such as cancer, MS, trauma, joint pain, and other conditions that provide chronic pain for those who are diagnosed. I also work along with women who are starting to approach middle age and older, those who aren't as confident about their bodies as they were ten years ago. I have enough personal knowledge of what immobility, extreme physical pain and growing older are all about, along with the emotional and mental challenges that we as women face in our society. I wanted to make sure that the knowledge I had could be shared with others and maybe provide the same gesture that Hope provided me all those years ago.

I found while learning about myself and teaching my

classes that all women are faced with the limitations thrust upon our sex by society. We may not be young enough, we might have wrinkles on our face, we might have a different body than we had in our prime, and there is also the discrimination of being an older adult. There is pressure put upon women to act a certain way based on our age and standards for beauty that don't seem to include those women that are older. It's been brought upon by years and years of people accepting the norms and ideas that are far outdated, but that doesn't mean that those molds can be broken. However, we can choose to see and project ourselves in a brighter more positive and radiant light. We can be the examples to lead other women walking behind us and alongside us on this positive and empowering path.

My classes consist of all of my accreditations, and I make sure that I use my knowledge to tailor classes to an individual's personal needs. I want to bring back the joy of movement and music into their lives in whatever capacity they need. I don't expect my clients to be accepting of my help right away; sometimes, the exercises I work them through are hard and many people have asked to stop because they don't think they'd be able to continue. I use their feedback to rework and change my routine in order to make them feel comfortable and safe in my classes. The last thing I ever want my students to think is that I don't care about them and that I just care about the message I'm spreading. For me, my messages and my goals for my clients work in tandem. They need to know that they should be celebrated for their work to get well and supported if they're having a tough time. There should be no shame between me or my clients; we are all working towards the same thing. I bring my heart and knowledge into helping every student. I want my classes to be a joy for them and to celebrate each milestone no matter how great or small.

My goal is for all of us to reclaim our power and gratitude for life. I want us all to experience an "aha" moment in order to escape from pain or the feeling of not being good enough, even if only for moments in time. I want us to break out of the prison of our limitations and see our lives through the new prism of hope and peace and joy. I end all my sessions the very same way with the quote, "Reach for the stars, for anything is possible." This helps to remind my students that they are strong enough to reach for what they might, at first, see as unattainable. Through my classes, I hope to tell them that quote and for them to realize that they've made it to their proverbial stars and have reached what they didn't believe could be possible.

The mind is a powerful thing. It connects us to the world around us and helps our body to process all sorts of stimuli. However, I feel that it should be seen as a healing tool. Changing our minds on something that we're so set on can be a powerful tool to help us move forward past a rough experience. Even if we physically are unable to perform certain movements, the joy and freedom that movement and music bring us can be used as a holistic extension to help us embrace the changes in our lives, to release us from our self-imposed prisons, and to see the light that a little shift of a prism can shine into our lives in a positive and healing way.

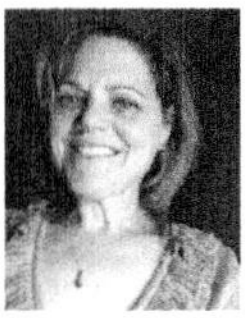

About Nancy Cashman

Nancy is an all around wellness enthusiast and teacher. She is accredited in several types of yoga as well BalletBeFit, Reiki Level 2, Meditation and High Impact Aerobics. In 2018, Nancy founded ZenAgain, LLC, a wellness organization that encompasses all of her knowledge and passion in wellness and Zen, and that is singularly committed to helping others find their own path to total mind, body and spiritual wellness.

Nancy is especially dedicated to helping those that are dealing with critical illness, pain and anxiety, and to helping enable women who are facing issues with the aging process to feel empowered in accessing their own mind-body connection to navigate their way to a sense of peace, calm and wellbeing. Nancy works with both individuals and in groups, and is known for her ability to connect to people and her genuine commitment to helping others achieve their individual wellness goals. Nancy's classes are tailored to each individual's needs in every class that she teaches.

Connect with Nancy at:

- nancy.cashman@yahoo.com